RESPIRATORY
CARE
REVIEW

RESPIRATORY CARE REVIEW

AN INTENSE LOOK AT RESPIRATORY CARE THROUGH CASE STUDIES

GARY A. KORZAN MS RRT

authorHOUSE®

AuthorHouse™
1663 Liberty Drive
Bloomington, IN 47403
www.authorhouse.com
Phone: 1-800-839-8640

Published by AuthorHouse   06/08/2012

ISBN: 978-1-4634-1817-5 (sc)
ISBN: 978-1-4634-1813-7 (e)

Library of Congress Control Number: 2011909779

CONTENTS

To all who engage
in
respiratory care education
and
clinical practice

INTRODUCTION

Dear Reader,

If you are about to embark on a journey through *Respiratory Care Review: An Intense Look at Respiratory Care through Case Studies*, chances are you are a respiratory care student in your final semester or quarter of your respiratory care program, or you are a recent graduate preparing for the NBRC CRT and RRT exams. Regardless of your current situation, this book was written specifically for you. Anxiety levels tend to run high as respiratory care students prepare for graduation or recent graduates prepare to take the NBRC exams. Hopefully, after working through the various case studies included in this book, you will feel more confident with your knowledge of respiratory care content and your ability to utilize your critical thinking skills.

Respiratory Care Review: An Intense Look at Respiratory Care through Case Studies would be best used as part of a formal respiratory care course, so that an instructor can evaluate your critical thinking skills in addition to probing for and correcting any respiratory care content weaknesses. However, the use of this book as part of a self-study strategy has the potential to achieve the same objectives. If you choose to use this book as part of a self-study strategy, having a qualified mentor would undoubtedly be very helpful.

It is important to note that the case studies included in this book have been abbreviated in order to focus on certain aspects of the highlighted cardiopulmonary conditions. Diagnostic test results not included in the discussion of a particular case study were either normal, or the diagnostic tests were not performed. Reference ranges for the various laboratory tests can be found at the end of this section. Since reference ranges vary from laboratory-to-laboratory, comparing the values with those used at your local medical centers might prove to be a useful exercise.

A variety of respiratory care texts commonly used in respiratory care programs throughout the country were consulted to formulate the discussion questions that accompany each case study. A list of these resources can be found at the end of this section.

Finally, the case studies are completely independent of each other and can be completed in any order.

I wholeheartedly wish each of you the best as you prepare for graduation or the NBRC exams.

Sincerely,
Gary A. Korzan MS RRT

REFERENCE RANGES

Complete Blood Count:

White Blood Cells $4.5\text{-}11.5 \times 10^3/mm^3$

Red Blood Cells $4.6\text{-}6.2 \times 10^6/mm^3$ (M) $4.2\text{-}5.4 \times 10^6/mm^3$ (F)

Hemoglobin   13.5-16.5 g/dL (M) 12.0-15.0 g/dL (F)

Hematocrit   40-54% (M) 38-47% (F)

Platelets $140\text{-}440 \times 10^3/mm^3$

Chemistry Profile:

Na^+ 137-147 mEq/L

K^+ 3.5-4.8 mEq/L

Cl^- 98-105 mEq/L

CO_2 25-33 mEq/L

Glucose   70-105 mg/dL

Blood Urea Nitrogen   7-20 mg/dL

Creatinine   0.7-1.3 mg/dL

Albumin   3.5-5.0 g/dL

Mg^{2+} 1.8-2.4 mg/dL

Cardiac Profile:

Creatine Kinase   39-308 U/L (M) 26-192 U/L (F)

Creatine Kinase-MB   0.5-3.6 ng/mL

Troponin   < 0 .1 ng/mL

B-type Natriuretic Peptide (BNP)   < 100 pg/mL

Coagulation Profile:

International Normalized Ratio (INR)   2.0-3.0 therapeutic range

Prothrombin Time (PT)   12-15 seconds

Activated Partial Thromboplastin Time (PTT)   24-32 seconds

Digoxin: 0.8-2.0 ng/mL

D-dimer: < 250 ng/mL

REFERENCES

Des Jardins, T. (2008). *Cardiopulmonary anatomy and physiology: Essentials of Respiratory Care* (5th ed.). Clifton Park, NY: Delmar Cengage Learning.

Des Jardins, T. & Burton, G. G. (2011). *Clinical manifestations and assessment of respiratory disease* (6th ed.). St. Louis, MO: Mosby.

Gardenhire, D. S. (2008). *Rau's respiratory care pharmacology* (7th ed.). St. Louis, MO: Mosby.

Pilbeam, S. P. & Cairo, J. M. (2006). *Mechanical ventilation: Physiological and clinical applications* (4th ed.). St. Louis, MO: Mosby

Walsh, B. K., Czervinske, M. P., & DiBlasi, R. M (2010). *Perinatal and pediatric respiratory care* (3rd ed.). St. Louis, MO: Saunders.

Wilkins, R. L., Dexter, F. R., & Heuer, A. J. (2010). *Clinical assessment in respiratory care* (6th ed.). St. Louis, MO: Mosby.

Wilkins, R. L., Stoller, J. K., & Kacmarek, R. M. (2009). *Egan's fundamentals of respiratory care* (9th ed.). St. Louis, MO: Mosby.

CASE STUDY 1

LARYNGOTRACHEOBRONCHITIS (LTB)/CROUP

CASE STUDY INTRODUCTION

The parents of RD were awakened by the sound of a barking cough and crying coming from the bedroom of their 19-month-old son. Since RD had been previously diagnosed with reactive airway disease (RAD), they administered an albuterol aerosol treatment to RD for what they determined to be audible wheezes. Since no relief in symptoms was observed following the aerosol treatment, they decided to transport RD to the local emergency department for evaluation.

INITIAL ASSESSMENT

Age: 19 months
Weight: 23 lbs (10.5 kg)
Heart Rate: 144 bpm
Respiratory Rate: 32 bpm
S_pO_2: 90% (room air)
Temperature: 37.0° C
Breath Sounds: audible inspiratory/expiratory stridor at rest (increased with crying), diminished breath sounds throughout all lung fields
Chest/Abdominal Inspection: mild suprasternal retractions
Cough/Sputum: strong, barking, congested, nonproductive
Level of Consciousness: alert
General Appearance/Behavior: active, occasional crying (crying increased following cough)
Medical/Surgical History: RAD
Current Medications: albuterol, budesonide
Allergies: amoxicillin

DIAGNOSTIC RESULTS

Laboratory: flu-negative, respiratory syncytial virus (RSV)-negative

Chest X-ray: "steeple point" narrowing of the upper airway

Lateral Neck X-ray: haziness in subglottic area

TREATMENT

racemic epinephrine 0.5 mL/3.0 mL normal saline aerosol treatment
dexamethasone 6 mg PO

COMMENTS

RD cried throughout the aerosol treatment. Halfway through the treatment, RD coughed and expectorated a large amount of thick, clear sputum. The stridor decreased significantly as the treatment progressed, and the cough sounded less harsh and congested. RD's heart rate increased from 144 to 156 bpm, and his respiratory rate decreased from 32 to 28 bpm. The skin under the aerosol mask blanched during the aerosol treatment which caused RD's parents to become momentarily alarmed. Within a few minutes following the aerosol treatment, RD was sleeping in his mother's arms.

An hour after receiving the ordered treatments, RD was alert and active. A mild inspiratory stridor was audible with crying. RD's cough, although still harsh, had significantly improved since the initial assessment. RD's vital signs were all within normal limits. The decision was made to discharge RD.

CASE DISCUSSION

1. List the pathologic or structural changes that are associated with croup?

2. Why is "laryngotracheobronchitis" a more appropriate term for croup?

3. What normal anatomical features of an infant's or small child's airway provide an additive effect in the airway obstruction associated with croup?

4. Why is it useful to assess the degree of stridor while a patient is at rest?

5. What is the significance of expiratory stridor?

6. As this case illustrates, stridor can be misinterpreted as wheezes. What clinical assessment procedure can be performed to confirm the presence of stridor?

7. How do retractions develop? Why are infants and younger children likely to have retractions when experiencing significant respiratory difficulty?

8. What explanation would you have provided to RD's parents for the lack of a positive therapeutic response to the albuterol aerosol treatment they administered to RD at home?

9. What kind of drug is racemic epinephrine? Why is racemic epinephrine indicated for the treatment of croup?

10. What was the likely reason for the sudden expectoration of a large amount of sputum halfway through the racemic epinephrine aerosol treatment?

11. Were any side effects observed during the administration of the racemic epinephrine that warranted the discontinuation of the aerosol treatment?

12. To prevent any unnecessary alarm by RD's parents, what explanation would you have provided to explain the blanching of the skin under the aerosol mask during the administration of the racemic epinephrine aerosol treatment?

13. Were there any signs that the racemic epinephrine was being effective during the aerosol treatment?

14. What kind of drug is dexamethasone? Why is it commonly administered along with a racemic epinephrine aerosol treatment for the treatment of croup?

15. If supplemental oxygen had been indicated for RD, which oxygen delivery device would you have used?

16. Was the lateral neck X-ray indicated in this case?

17. List the etiological factors and assessment findings associated with croup and epiglottitis.

CROUP	EPIGLOTTITIS

18. What precautions need to be taken during the assessment of a patient suspected of having epiglottitis?

19. How is the treatment for epiglottitis different than the treatment for croup?

20. RD cried throughout the aerosol treatment. Comments are often made by parents and clinicians that the patient receives more medication when crying. Do you agree or disagree with these comments?

21. What is the preferential method for administering an aerosol treatment to an infant or younger child (mouthpiece, mask, or blow-by)?

22. Antibiotics were not administered to RD during his emergency department visit, nor were they prescribed prior to discharge. Was this an oversight on behalf of the physician?

23. Do you believe it is in the scope of respiratory care for respiratory therapists to assess a patient for pain?

24. Were there any clues that RD was experiencing pain?

25. Do you agree with the physician's decision to discharge RD? What potential assessment findings would have indicated that RD required admission to the hospital?

CASE STUDY 2

CONGESTIVE HEART FAILURE (CHF)

CASE INTRODUCTION

RK was transported to the local emergency department after developing a sudden onset of shortness of breath. An EMS paramedic recorded RK's S_pO_2 at 65% on room air upon arrival at his residence. RK was administered supplemental oxygen via a non-rebreathing mask at 15 L/min while being transported to the emergency department.

INITIAL ASSESSMENT

Age: 69-years-old
Height: 5' 8"
Weight: 170 lbs. (77 kg)
Heart Rate: 132 bpm
Respiratory Rate: 44 bpm
Blood Pressure: 215/116 mm Hg
S_pO_2: 81% (non-rebreathing mask at 15 L/min)
Temperature: 37.0° C
Breath Sounds: wheezes and rhonchi (upper lobes), crackles (lower lobes)
Chest/Abdominal Inspection: expiratory accessory muscle use
Cough/Sputum: strong, congested, productive/ large amounts of frothy, pink-tinged sputum
Level of Consciousness: alert/oriented x 3
General Appearance/Behavior: diaphoretic, jugular venous distention (JVD), pedal edema, anxious
Medical/Surgical History: chronic obstructive pulmonary disease (COPD), coronary artery disease (CAD), CHF, myocardial infarction (MI), coronary artery bypass graft (CABG) surgery, repeat CABG for coronary artery aneurysm, mitral valve replacement, automated implantable cardioverter defibrillator (AICD) insertion, cardiac catherization with stent placement, depression
Social History: smoker 1/2 PPD (1/2 to 2 PPD x 51 years)
Current Medications: aspirin, digoxin, lisinopril, spironolactone, carvedilol, escitalopram oxalate
Allergies: latex

INITIAL TREATMENT

CPAP (continuous positive airway pressure) +10 cm H_2O 60% O_2
methylprednisolone 125 mg IV
aspirin 162 mg PO
furosemide 40 mg IV
metoprolol tartrate 5 mg IV
nitroglycerin paste 1"
albuterol/ipratropium bromide unit dose aerosol treatment x 1
albuterol 2.5 mg unit dose aerosol treatment x 2

COMMENTS

RK tolerated the CPAP well. The wheezes and rhonchi improved with the CPAP therapy, and RK's work of breathing was significantly reduced. Crackles were auscultated in both lower lobes. RK's S_pO_2 increased to 94%, but his respiratory rate remained between 40 and 45 bpm. Over a 15-minute period after the initiation of treatment, RK's blood pressure and heart rate decreased to 150/88 mm Hg and 90 bpm, respectively.

CASE DISCUSSION

1. Based on the initial treatment strategy, to which cardiopulmonary condition(s) was the treatment being directed?

2. What were the indications for the use of CPAP?

3. Describe the specific physiologic effects of CPAP.

4. Why would an oronasal CPAP mask be preferred in this case rather than a nasal CPAP mask?

5. How effective was the CPAP therapy for RK?

6. Were the bronchodilator aerosol treatments and methylprednisolone indicated?

7. How would you have administered the aerosol treatments while RK was receiving CPAP therapy with an oronasal mask?

DIAGNOSTIC RESULTS

Chest X-ray: cardiomegaly, pulmonary venous hypertension and congestion, bilateral fluffy infiltrates, bilateral pleural effusions (R > L)

Complete Blood Count:
White Blood Cells = 11.3 x 10^3/mm^3
Red Blood Cells = 5.05 x 10^6/mm^3
Hemoglobin = 16.1 g/dL
Hematocrit = 48.3%
Platelets = 218 x 10^3/mm^3

Chemistry Profile:
Na^+ = 139 mEq/L
K^+ = 4.0 mEq/L
Cl^- = 102 mEq/L
CO_2 = 25 mEq/L
Glucose = 159 mg/dL
Blood Urea Nitrogen = 25 mg/dL
Creatinine = 1.2 mg/dL
Albumin = 2.0 g/dL
Mg^{2+} = 2.1 mg/dL

Cardiac Profile:
Creatine Kinase: 45 U/L
Troponin: 0.04 ng/mL
B-type Natriuretic Peptide (BNP): 725 pg/mL

Digoxin: 0.67 ng/mL

ABG: (CPAP +10 cm H_2O 60% O_2-one hour after CPAP initiated)
Hb = 16.1 g/dL
pH = 7.19
$PaCO_2$ = 74 mm Hg
PaO_2 = 100 mm Hg
SaO_2 = 100%
HCO_3^- = 27 mEq/L
BE = 0 mEq/L
CaO_2 = 21.9 Vol%

ABG Interpretation: _____

COMMENTS

At the time the ABG was drawn, RK reported that he was having a difficult time breathing. His respiratory rate was still between 40 and 45 bpm. After consulting with RK and his wife, the decision for intubation and mechanical ventilation was made by the emergency department physician. Following the induction of etomidate and succinylcholine, the emergency department resident successfully intubated RK with an 8.0 mm endotracheal tube. The initial ventilator settings were: AC 12 600 mL 50% O_2 PEEP +10 cm H_2O. A propofol drip was initiated to maintain sedation. A blood pressure check ten minutes after the propofol drip was started revealed a blood pressure of 68/40 mm Hg. The propofol drip rate was decreased, and RK's blood pressure gradually recovered to 110/65 mm Hg.

DIAGNOSTIC RESULTS

Chest X-ray: tip of endotracheal tube 3.5 cm above carina, cardiomegaly, pulmonary venous hypertension and congestion, bilateral fluffy infiltrates, bilateral pleural effusions (R > L)

ABG: (AC 12 600 mL 50% O_2 PEEP +10 cm H_2O) (total respiratory rate = 12 bpm)
Hb = 15.8 g/dL
pH = 7.32
$PaCO_2$ = 50 mm Hg
PaO_2 = 92 mm Hg
SaO_2 = 98%
HCO_3^- = 25 mEq/L
BE = $^-$1 mEq/L
CaO_2 = 21.0 Vol%

ABG Interpretation: _____

Ventilation Mechanics:
Plateau Pressure (P_{PLAT}): 32 cm H_2O
Static Lung Compliance (C_S): 27 mL/cm H_2O
Airway Resistance (R_{AW}): 12 cm H_2O/L/sec

COMMENTS

Ventilator settings were adjusted to: AC 14 600 mL 50% O_2 PEEP +10 cm H_2O.

DIAGNOSTIC RESULTS

ABG: (AC 14 600 mL 50% O_2 PEEP +10 cm H_2O) (total respiratory rate = 14 bpm)

Hb = 15.5 g/dL

pH = 7.42

$PaCO_2$ = 38 mm Hg

PaO_2 = 97 mm Hg

SaO_2 = 98%

HCO_3^- = 24 mEq/L

BE = 0 mEq/L

CaO_2 = 20.6 Vol%

ABG Interpretation: _____

CASE DISCUSSION

8. Do you think bi-level noninvasive positive pressure ventilation (NPPV) would have been a viable option to intubation and mechanical ventilation in this case?

9. Were the initial ventilator settings and subsequent changes appropriate?

10. What does the BNP measure? What was the significance of the 725 pg/mL BNP?

11. What kind of medication is digoxin? What is the normal therapeutic range for digoxin? Was RK's digoxin level within the therapeutic range?

12. RK's P_{PLAT}, C_S, and R_{AW} were all determined while RK was sedated following intubation. What are the normal ranges for each of these measurements? How did RK's values compare to the normal ranges for each of these measurements?

13. How would you have expected RK's P_{PLAT}, C_S, and R_{AW} values to change as he diuresed following the administration of furosemide?

14. What is the normal range for albumin? Do you believe RK's albumin level played a role in his CHF exacerbation?

15. Excessive PEEP can result in a significant decrease in blood pressure. What potential complication(s) might have occurred in this case if the PEEP had been decreased to +5 cm H_2O when RK became hypotensive secondary to the propofol administration?

16. Explain the difference between interstitial pulmonary edema and alveolar pulmonary edema.

17. What causes the wheezes (often audible) when a patient experiences interstitial pulmonary edema? What causes the rhonchi and crackles when a patient experiences alveolar pulmonary edema?

18. Are bronchodilator or corticosteroid medications indicated for the treatment of pulmonary edema?

19. What does the pulmonary capillary wedge pressure (PCWP) measure? What is the normal PCWP range? If a pulmonary artery catheter is inserted, but the balloon is not inflated, how can the PCWP be estimated?

20. List at least four pathologic or structural changes that can increase the pulmonary venous and pulmonary capillary pressures, which in turn can lead to the development of cardiogenic pulmonary edema.

21. Define ventricular preload. How is cardiac output related to the ventricular preload? How is the best preload approximation determined?

22. Define ventricular afterload. How is ventricular afterload related to the systemic blood pressure?

23. Define cardiac contractility. How is cardiac output related to cardiac contractility?

24. How can ventricular preload, ventricular afterload, and cardiac contractility play a role in the development of cardiogenic pulmonary edema?

25. While surprisingly not occurring in this case, it is common for a severely hypoxic patient to show a metabolic acidosis component during ABG analysis. What causes the metabolic acidosis in a hypoxic situation?

26. How is the anion gap used in a clinical situation involving metabolic acidosis? How is the anion gap calculated? What is the normal anion gap range? Calculate RK's anion gap.

27. Although not administered in this case, how can morphine sulfate be useful during a CHF exacerbation?

28. There are a wide variety of psychological and biochemical causes for depression. Why do you think depression would be a problem for RK? Do you think RK's depression and smoking habit were related?

COMMENTS

RK's condition gradually improved over a 24-hour period, and he was extubated. Two days later he was discharged. While receiving his discharge instructions and related patient education, RK stated that he had not taken his carvedilol (beta-blocker) for four days due to an unexpected delay with his mail order. RK's wife advised him that the delivery arrived the day after his admission to the hospital.

CASE STUDY 3

SMOKE INHALATION/THERMAL INJURY

CASE INTRODUCTION

HP was transported to a local emergency department after involvement in a house fire of unknown origin. HP was intoxicated and could not recall any events leading up to the fire. He only remembered waking up and trying to exit the house at which time he received multiple burns over a large part of his upper body. He denied the need for treatment, but was convinced by family members to be transported by EMS personnel to the emergency department. He was transported with supplemental oxygen via a non-rebreathing mask at 15 L/min. EMS personnel reported that the house was completely destroyed by the fire.

INITIAL ASSESSMENT

Age: 32-years-old
Height: 5' 8"
Weight: 180 lbs. (82 kg)
Heart Rate: 114 bpm
Respiratory Rate: 24 bpm
Blood Pressure: 164/78 mm Hg
S$_p$O$_2$: 98% (non-rebreathing mask at > 15 L/min)
Temperature: 37.6° C
Breath Sounds: severely diminished throughout all lung fields, hoarse voice
Chest/Abdominal Inspection: expiratory accessory muscle use
Cough/Sputum: fair, congested, productive/large amounts of thick, black, sooty sputum
Level of Consciousness: alert/oriented x 1
General Appearance/Behavior: intoxicated, passively cooperative
Skin: first and second degree burns over face, head, upper chest, upper back, shoulders, and arms (total estimate 45% using the "rule of nines"); singed hair on head and face; soot over face and head
Eyes: burning sensation in both eyes
Medical/Surgical History: hypertension
Social History: smoker 1-2 PPD x 14 years, ethyl alcohol (ETOH) abuse
Current Mediations: metoprolol succinate
Allergies: no known allergies

INITIAL TREATMENT

oxygen via non-rebreathing mask at > 15 L/min
Ringer's lactate IV fluids at 1000 mL/hr (2 IV lines)
wet dressing applications to burns
irrigation of eyes

DIAGNOSTIC RESULTS

Chest X-ray: no infiltrates, pulmonary vasculature and cardiac silhouette appear normal

ABG: (non-rebreathing mask at > 15 L/min)
Hb = 16.0 g/dL
pH = 7.36
$PaCO_2$ = 38 mm Hg
PaO_2 = 106 mm Hg
SaO_2 = 99%
HCO_3^- = 21 mEq/L
BE = -4 mEq/L
CaO_2 = 21.5 Vol%

ABG Interpretation: _____

CO-oximetry:
COHb = 25.7%

ETOH: 0.345 g/dL

COMMENTS

While awaiting arrival of a helicopter transport team to transport HP to the regional burn center, HP became agitated and developed respiratory distress. (It was estimated by EMS personnel that HP had suffered his injuries about 1 1/2 hours prior to arrival at the emergency department.) Upon arrival, the transport team physician opted to intubate HP prior to transport. Ketamine and succinylcholine were administered to HP, and three attempts to intubate with an 8.0 mm endotracheal tube were unsuccessful. The physician reported extensive airway edema. A hospital anesthesiologist was called to assist, and HP was successfully intubated with a 7.0 mm endotracheal tube. HP was then transported without further delay to the regional burn center.

CASE DISCUSSION

1. Which of the assessment details indicated that HP had suffered airway thermal injuries and/or smoke inhalation injuries?

2. Unless steam is inhaled, why are thermal injuries typically limited to the upper airway? Why is the inhalation of steam an exception?

3. List the pathologic or structural changes associated with upper airway thermal injury.

4. List the pathologic or structural changes associated with lower airway smoke inhalation injury.

5. Was the decision to intubate HP prior to transport to the regional burn center appropriate?

6. Would you have agreed with a decision to intubate HP immediately upon his arrival to the emergency department?

7. What effect did the difficult intubation likely have on HP's condition?

8. Were there any clues in the ABG results suggesting that HP had experienced hypoxia prior to receiving supplemental oxygen?

9. What was the significance of the CO-oximetry results? Were the results adequately addressed in the initial treatment plan?

10. Could the CaO_2 as calculated by the ABG analyzer be useful in determining oxygen delivery to the tissues in this case?

11. Did the fact that HP smoked 1 to 2 PPD have any bearing on the CO-oximetry results?

12. The documentation reported that HP was receiving 100% oxygen while receiving supplemental oxygen via a non-rebreathing mask at 15 L/min. Was this documentation appropriate?

13. Two intravenous lines were inserted, and Ringer's lactate solution was infused into both lines at a rate of 1000 mL/hr. What was the rationale for this action? What possible deleterious effect(s) can occur following the rapid infusion of intravenous fluids?

14. What would have been your initial volume ventilation ventilator settings? What adjustments would you have made for a high plateau pressure (> 30-35 cm H_2O)?

15. List at least four factors that would have contributed to an increased airway resistance while HP was receiving mechanical ventilation. How could each of the four factors have been addressed in an effort to reduce the airway resistance?

16. How would you have expected lung compliance to be affected by the smoke inhalation injuries HP received?

17. The burning of plastics and other synthetic materials can produce smoke containing cyanide. How does cyanide poisoning affect tissue oxygenation? Why is lactic acidosis associated with cyanide poisoning?

18. Was HP a candidate for hyperbaric oxygen therapy? How is hyperbaric oxygen therapy helpful in a smoke inhalation/thermal injury case?

19. Why would endotracheal tube cuff pressure or tracheostomy tube cuff pressure management have been important in this case?

20. How should a respiratory therapist prepare for extubation in this type of case?

21. What would a post-extubation respiratory care plan likely include?

CASE STUDY 4

GUILLAIN-BARRE SYNDROME

CASE INTRODUCTION

DM presented to the emergency department complaining of increasing weakness in his legs over a 24-hour period. He stated that he had been feeling fine until he started to feel a tingling sensation and weakness in his legs the previous day. He did, however, state that he had a bad case of the flu within the past month that kept him home from work for a period of five days. DM was employed as a carpenter for a construction company at the time of this illness. Based on DM's history and clinical presentation, he was admitted to the ICU with a preliminary diagnosis of Guillain-Barre syndrome. A neurology consult was ordered by the emergency department physician.

INITIAL ASSESSMENT

Age: 53-years-old
Height: 6' 0"
Weight: 176 lbs. (80 kg)
Heart Rate: 68 bpm
Respiratory Rate: 20 bpm
Blood Pressure: 120/76 mm Hg
S_pO_2: 98% (room air)
Temperature: 37.0° C
Breath Sounds: clear throughout all lung fields
Chest/Abdominal Inspection: normal
Cough/Sputum: strong, dry, nonproductive
Level of Consciousness: alert/oriented x 3
General Appearance/Behavior: calm, resting comfortably
Neuromuscular: generalized weakness in legs, able to walk independently (slowly)
Medical/Surgical History: appendectomy
Social History: non-smoker
Current Medications: none
Allergies: no known allergies

DIAGNOSTIC RESULTS

Chest X-ray: no infiltrates, pulmonary vasculature and cardiac silhouette appear normal

COMMENTS

Between the time of admission to the ICU and the time seen by the consulted neurologist (approximately two hours), DM's leg weakness had increased to the point he could no longer stand without assistance. The neurologist confirmed the diagnosis of Guillain-Barre syndrome based on DM's clinical presentation and history. The ICU intensivist ordered bedside maximum inspiratory pressure (MIP) and vital capacity (VC) tests to be administered by the respiratory department staff every two hours.

DIAGNOSTIC RESULTS

TIME	MIP (cm H_2O)	VC (L)
1000	-50	4.3
1200	-45	3.7
1400	-40	3.0
1600	-30	2.2
1800	-20	1.8
2000	-15	1.0

ABG: (2000-nasal cannula at 3 L/min)
Hb = 13.5 g/dL
pH = 7.30
$PaCO_2$ = 60 mm Hg
PaO_2 = 62 mm Hg
SaO_2 = 91%
HCO_3^- = 29 mEq/L
BE = 3 mEq/L
CaO_2 = 16.6 Vol%

ABG Interpretation: _____

ASSESSMENT

(2000)
Heart Rate: 100 bpm
Respiratory Rate: 32 bpm
Blood Pressure: 136/90 mm Hg
S_pO_2: 91% (nasal cannula at 3 L/min)
Temperature: 37.0° C
Breath Sounds: clear (upper lobes), diminished (lower lobes)
Chest/Abdominal Inspection: inspiratory accessory muscle use
Cough/Sputum: weak, dry, nonproductive
Level of Consciousness: alert/oriented x 3
General Appearance/Behavior: anxious
Neuromuscular: lower extremity paralysis, severe upper extremity weakness, able to lift head off pillow, dysphagia

COMMENTS

Based on the ABG, MIP, and VC results, as well as DM's clinical assessment at 2000, the decision to intubate DM was made following a brief discussion with DM and his family. DM was successfully intubated with an 8.0 mm endotracheal tube on the first attempt by the respiratory therapist following the administration of midazolam. The initial ventilator settings were: AC 12 650 mL 50% O_2 PEEP +5 cm H_2O. Plans were made to transfer DM to a local parternship hospital early the next morning for plasmapheresis therapy.

DIAGNOSTIC RESULTS
ABG: (AC 12 650 mL 50% O_2 PEEP +5 cm H_2O) (total respiratory rate = 12 bpm)
Hb = 13.0 g/dL
pH = 7.48
$PaCO_2$ = 30 mm Hg
PaO_2 = 240 mm Hg
SaO_2 = 100%
HCO_3^- = 22 mEq/L
BE = -2 mEq/L
CaO_2 = 18.1 Vol%

ABG Interpretation: _____

Chest X-ray: endotracheal tube positioned 3 cm above carina, bilateral lower lobe atelectasis

COMMENTS
Ventilator settings were adjusted to: AC 10 650 mL 30% O_2 PEEP +8 cm H_2O. A dexmedetomidine drip was initiated to maintain sedation overnight.

DIAGNOSTIC RESULTS
ABG: (AC 10 650 mL 30% O_2 PEEP +8 cm H_2O) (total respiratory rate = 10 bpm)
Hb = 12.8 g/dL
pH = 7.39
$PaCO_2$ = 42 mm Hg
PaO_2 = 93 mm Hg
SaO_2 = 97%
HCO_3^- = 25 mEq/L
BE = 0 mEq/L
CaO_2 = 17.0 Vol%

ABG Interpretation: _____

Ventilation Mechanics:
Plateau Pressure (P_{PLAT}): 17 cm H_2O
Static Lung Compliance (C_S): 72 mL/cm H_2O
Airway Resistance (R_{AW}): 5 cm H_2O/L/sec

ASSESSMENT
Heart Rate: 68 bpm
Respiratory Rate: 10 bpm
Blood Pressure: 110/58 mm Hg
S$_p$O$_2$: 97% (AC 10 650 mL 30% O$_2$ PEEP +8 cm H$_2$O)
Temperature: 37.0° C
Breath Sounds: clear (upper lobes), diminished (lower lobes)
Chest/Abdominal Inspection: normal
Cough/Sputum: none
Level of Consciousness: appropriately sedated

COMMENTS
DM was transferred to a local partnership hospital by ground transport without incident the following morning for plasmapheresis therapy as planned. DM required ventilator support for an additional fifteen days before being extubated. The endotracheal tube was changed on the tenth day of mechanical ventilation due to a persistent cuff leak. The insertion of a tracheostomy tube was put on hold at the time the endotracheal tube was changed due to significant improvements observed in DM's neuromuscular status. He was eventually transferred to a skilled nursing unit within the same hospital for intensive physical therapy for a period of one month. DM returned to his job three weeks after being discharged from the skilled nursing unit.

CASE DISCUSSION
1. List the pathologic or structural changes associated with Guillain-Barre syndrome.

2. What causes Guillain-Barre syndrome?

3. What was the significance of the flu that DM had prior to the development of Guillain-Barre syndrome?

4. What diagnostic test(s) could have been performed to provide more supportive evidence for the diagnosis of Guillain-Barre syndrome?

5. Was the rate of paralysis development consistent with Guillain-Barre syndrome?

6. How would you describe DM's respiratory status at the time of admission to the emergency department?

7. What does a MIP test actually measure? What is an adequate MIP value? Why did the ICU intensivist order the monitoring of DM's MIP values?

8. Using a VC measurement <15 mL/kg (IBW) as an indication for ventilatory support, at what time did DM's VC measurement indicate the need for ventilatory support?

9. What evidence did the ICU intensivist likely present to DM and his family when discussing the need for intubation and mechanical ventilation?

10. Do you think bi-level noninvasive positive pressure ventilation (NPPV) would have been a viable option to intubation and mechanical ventilation in this case?

11. The ABG prior to intubation was drawn at 2000. Were there any indications from the MIP/VC results to have the ABG drawn at an earlier time?

12. What patient assessment factors needed to be monitored along with the ABG and MIP/VC measurements when determining indications for ventilatory support?

13. What assessments are performed to ensure that the endotracheal tube is properly positioned in a patient's airway? How is correct endotracheal tube placement confirmed?

14. Were the initial ventilator settings and subsequent changes appropriate?

15. What was the indication for increasing the PEEP from +5 cm H_2O to +8 cm H_2O? How would this change have been evaluated for effectiveness?

16. What is your evaluation of DM's P_{PLAT}, C_S, and R_{AW} measurements?

17. Why was the persistent endotracheal tube cuff leak a concern?

18. In addition to ventilatory failure, what are the potential respiratory complications associated with Guillain-Barre syndrome?

19. What are the advantages and disadvantages of a tracheostomy tube compared to an endotracheal tube for a patient requiring long-term mechanical ventilation?

20. What is the purpose of plasmapheresis therapy in the treatment of Guillain-Barre syndrome? What other treatment options are available for Guillain-Barre syndrome?

21. List the pathologic or structural changes associated with myasthenia gravis.

22. What causes myasthenia gravis?

23. In addition to ventilatory failure, what are the potential respiratory complications associated with myasthenia gravis?

24. Describe the edrophonium (Tensilon) test.

25. What is the purpose of plasmapheresis therapy in the treatment of myasthenia gravis? What other treatment options are available for myasthenia gravis?

CASE STUDY 5

ASTHMA

CASE INTRODUCTION

SK was on the third and last day of a weekend Boy Scout camp out when symptoms of his asthma started to become a nuisance. SK's asthma was generally well-controlled, and exacerbations were typically few in number throughout the year. SK attributed his symptoms to the smoke he incidentally inhaled from the campfires the previous night. Throughout the day, he checked his peak flow rates as he had been instructed and used his albuterol MDI as prescribed. By evening, his peak flow rate had decreased from 85% to 60% of his personal best peak flow rate, and he was becoming more symptomatic. SK notified his scout leader, and he was driven to a local 40-bed hospital which had treated many Boy Scouts and Girl Scouts using the campground over the years. SK's parents, who lived about two hours away from the campground, were notified by the scout leader prior to the transport, and were given frequent updates while SK was at the hospital.

INITIAL ASSESSMENT

Age: 12-years-old
Height: 5' 2"
Weight: 86 lbs. (39 kg)
Heart Rate: 115 bpm
Respiratory Rate: 28 bpm
Blood Pressure: 110/70 mm Hg
S_pO_2: 89% (room air)
Temperature: 37.5° C
Breath Sounds: inspiratory/expiratory wheezes and diminished throughout all lung fields
Chest/Abdominal Inspection: expiratory accessory muscle use
Pulsus Paradoxus: not detected by radial pulse palpation
Cough/Sputum: strong, wheezy, productive/moderate amounts of thick, white secretions
Level of Consciousness: alert/oriented x 3
General Appearance/Behavior: anxious, tripod position
Medical/Surgical History: reactive airway disease/asthma (since 2-years-old)
Current Medications: montelukast, albuterol MDI
Allergies: various pollens and mold spores, no medication allergies

INITIAL TREATMENT

albuterol/ipratropium bromide unit dose aerosol treatment x 1
albuterol 2.5 mg unit dose aerosol treatment x 2
prednisone 60 mg PO

ASSESSMENT/TREATMENT RECORD

(Personal Best Peak Flow Rate (PEFR) = 300 L/min)

TIME	HR (bpm)	RR (bpm)	S_pO_2	BREATH SOUNDS	ACC. MUSCLES	PRE-PEFR (L/min)	MED	POST-PEFR (L/min)
1830	110	28	89% (RA)	I/E WH-DIM	Y	140	albuterol/ ipratropium bromide	150
1850	115	28	92% (RA)	E WH-DIM	Y	150	albuterol	210
1910	130	24	94% (RA)	E WH	N	200	albuterol	220

DIAGNOSTIC RESULTS

Chest X-ray: (1930) mild hyperinflation, no infiltrates

ASSESSMENT/TREATMENT RECORD

TIME	HR (bpm)	RR (bpm)	S_pO_2	BREATH SOUNDS	ACC. MUSCLES	PRE-PEFR (L/min)	MED	POST-PEFR (L/min)
2000	112	24	94% (RA)	E WH (End-exh)	N	200	-	-
2010	-	-	-	-	-	-	albuterol 2 puffs	-
2020	110	20	96% (RA)	E-WH (End-exh)	N	-	-	230

COMMENTS

SK was monitored for another 40 minutes and then discharged after a final assessment by the emergency department physician. SK stated that he was breathing much better and that he was anxious to get back to the campground for the last night of the camp out. SK's discharge instructions recommended that he continue to follow his current asthma plan and to follow up with his physician after returning home. SK was discharged with four, 60 mg doses of prednisone to be used over the next four days.

CASE DISCUSSION

1. How competent do you think SK was in managing his asthma using the asthma treatment plan that his physician designed for him?

2. The predicted PEFR for SK using the table supplied with the peak flow meter was 400 L/min. What was the value of SK knowing his personal best PEFR in this case?

3. How would you instruct a patient to determine his/her personal best PEFR?

4. Which assessment changes indicated that SK was having a positive response to the emergency department treatment plan? Were there any deleterious effects to the treatments SK received?

5. Why do you suppose the emergency department physician ordered the albuterol MDI treatment instead of a fourth albuterol 2.5 mg unit dose aerosol treatment?

6. Do you agree with the emergency department physician's decision to discharge SK?

7. Would you describe SK's asthma as being extrinsic, intrinsic, or a combination of the two?

8. During an asthma exacerbation, what three pathologic or structural changes lead to air trapping and hyperinflation? How are each of these three pathologic or structural changes addressed within a typical respiratory care plan for the treatment of asthma?

9. What causes pulsus paradoxus during a severe asthma exacerbation? What is the easiest method for assessing for pulsus paradoxus?

10. List at least three chest X-ray findings that indicate hyperinflation.

11. What chest palpation and percussion assessment findings are associated with an asthma exacerbation?

12. What is the significance of the tripod position that SK assumed?

13. What are some ominous signs that a patient having a severe asthma exacerbation requires intubation and mechanical ventilation?

14. How are the following pulmonary function measurements affected during an asthma exacerbation with significant air trapping?

	NORMAL	INCREASED	DECREASED
FVC			
FEV_1			
$FEV_{1\%}$			
PEFR			
RV			
ERV			
FRC			
TLC			
RV/TLC RATIO			

15. How are the FVC, FEV_1, and $FEV_{1\%}$ used to distinguish between obstructive and restrictive pulmonary defects?

16. What kind of drug is montelukast? Why is it commonly prescribed for patients with asthma?

17. How do corticosteroids affect the responsiveness of beta receptors in the airways to beta-adrenergic stimulation? Why is it beneficial to administer corticosteroids as soon as possible during an asthma exacerbation?

18. Outline the series of events that occur from the exposure to an antigen in a susceptible person to the development of an asthma exacerbation.

19. Why should asthmatics be educated about the early and late asthmatic responses to inhaled antigens?

20. List at least four factors that may cause a nocturnal asthmatic episode.

21. List at least two kinds of medications that can provoke an asthmatic episode.

22. When does an exercise-induced asthmatic episode typically occur?

23. List at least two weather-related causes of an asthmatic episode?

CASE STUDY 6

ACUTE MYOCARDIAL INFARCTION (AMI)

CASE INTRODUCTION

The wife of TL contacted EMS after finding her husband clutching his chest, sweating profusely, and experiencing severe shortness of breath. TL had just climbed a flight of stairs prior to the onset of his symptoms. TL was scheduled to have coronary artery bypass graft (CABG) and aortic valve replacement surgery the following week. EMS personnel transmitted TL's ECG to the emergency department, and an ST segment elevation myocardial infarction (STEMI) was quickly determined. The cardiac catherization team on call was notified, and a "STEMI Alert" was called at the hospital to prepare for TL's arrival to the emergency department.

INITIAL ASSESSMENT

Age: 65-years-old
Height: 5' 10"
Weight: 160 lbs. (73 kg)
Heart Rate: 60 bpm
Respiratory Rate: 32 bpm
Blood Pressure: 138/70 mm Hg
S_pO_2: 98% (non-rebreathing mask at 15 L/min)
Temperature: 37.2° C
Breath Sounds: severely diminished throughout all lung fields (decreased inspiratory efforts due to severe chest pain), crackles (lower lobes)
Chest/Abdominal Inspection: decreased chest expansion
Cough/Sputum: fair, moist, nonproductive
Level of Consciousness: alert/oriented x 3
General Appearance/Behavior: diaphoretic, gray, clutching chest, moaning, irritated by assessment questioning
Medical/Surgical History: chronic obstructive pulmonary disease (COPD), coronary artery disease (CAD), myocardial infarction (MI), congestive heart failure (CHF), end-stage renal disease (ESRD), dialysis, hypertension, severe aortic stenosis, chronic anemia, hyperlipidemia
Social History: smoker 1-2 PPD x 47 years
Current Medications: albuterol MDI, aspirin, tiotropium bromide, carvedilol, lisinopril, cinacalcet, nitroglycerin (sublingual tablets), rosuvastatin, sevelamer
Allergies: penicillin

INITIAL TREATMENT
aspirin 162 mg PO
nitroglycerin drip IV at 10 mcg/hr
lorazepam 1 mg IV
heparin 4380 U IV bolus (60 U/kg)
heparin drip IV (per protocol)
morphine sulfate 4 mg IV

COMMENTS
TL's clinical presentation was very poor on arrival to the emergency department. He was experiencing severe chest pain that radiated to his left arm and jaw, and his color was gray. Equipment was set up by a respiratory therapist for an imminent intubation. Over the next 45 minutes, the nitroglycerin drip was gradually increased from 10 mcg/hr to 60 mcg/hr with only minimal relief from the chest pain. The non-rebreathing mask was replaced with a 50% air entrainment mask. TL's blood pressure remained stable between 135-145/60-70 mm Hg.

DIAGNOSTIC RESULTS
ECG: STEMI

Chest X-ray: cardiomegaly, CHF

ABG: (50% air entrainment mask)
Hb = 8.9 g/dL
pH = 7.63
$PaCO_2$ = 34 mm Hg
PaO_2 = 202 mm Hg
SaO_2 = 100%
HCO_3^- = 35 mEq/L
BE = 13 mEq/L

ABG Interpretation: _____

Complete Blood Count:
White Blood Cells = 6.2 x 10^3/mm^3
Red Blood Cells = 2.76 x 10^6/mm^3
Hemoglobin = 8.7 g/dL
Hematocrit = 26.6%
Platelets = 377 x 10^3/mm^3

Chemistry Profile:
Na^+ = 133 mEq/L
K^+ = 4.0 mEq/L
Cl^- = 91 mEq/L
CO_2 = 33 mEq/L
Glucose = 109 mg/dL
Blood Urea Nitrogen = 26 mg/dL
Creatinine = 7.5 mg/dL
Albumin = 2.7 g/dL
Mg^{2+} = 1.9 mg/dL

Cardiac Profile:
Creatine Kinase: 480 U/L (NOTE: increased to 2056 U/L over 15-hour period)
Creatine Kinase-MB: 36 ng/mL (NOTE: increased to 255 ng/mL over 15-hour period)
Troponin: 0.35 ng/mL (NOTE: increased to > 80 ng/mL over 15-hour period)
B-type Natriuretic Peptide (BNP): 3261 pg/mL

Coagulation Profile:
International Normalized Ratio (INR): 1.20
Prothrombin Time (PT): 12.7 sec
Activated Partial Thromboplastin Time (PTT): 29.4 sec

COMMENTS

The F_IO_2 was decreased from 50% to 30% on the air entrainment mask, and TL was transported to the cardiac catherization lab. During the cardiac catherization procedure, the physician inserted a stent into TL's left anterior descending coronary artery (LAD) and initiated intra-aortic balloon counterpulsation (IABC) therapy to assist with cardiac pump function and to reduce myocardial ischemia. Shortly after the procedures, TL developed atrial fibrillation with a rapid ventricular rate which required three cardioversion attempts to return the irregular rhythm to a normal sinus rhythm. The physician opted to use propofol to sedate TL for the cardioversion and requested the assistance of a respiratory therapist for the "conscious sedation" procedure. TL required manual ventilation with a bag-valve mask resuscitator for approximately five minutes following the induction of the propofol. After fully awakening from the cardioversion, the 30% air entrainment mask was used to provide TL with supplemental oxygen. TL continued to have significant chest pain after the cardiac catherization, but the subjective pain level had decreased from a rating of 10 to a rating of 5. He was transported to the cardiac care unit (CCU) for further care.

CASE DISCUSSION

1. Why would TL's CABG and aortic valve replacement surgery have been considered very high-risk procedures even before the acute STEMI?

2. What significance does the elevated ST segment have in a STEMI?

3. What kind of drug is nitroglycerin? How is it helpful in the treatment of a STEMI?

4. What role does aspirin and heparin play in the treatment of a STEMI? Why would serial coagulation tests be ordered for TL?

5. What kind of drug is morphine sulfate? How is it helpful in the treatment of a STEMI?

6. Which lab values in the complete blood count supported TL's medical history for chronic anemia? Why was it important for the clinicians to be aware of this aspect of TL's medical history?

7. Which lab values were consistent with TL's medical history for chronic renal failure?

8. Why do the creatine kinase-MB and troponin serum levels increase following a myocardial infarction?

9. Did TL's albumin level likely play a role in his condition?

10. Calculate the arterial oxygen content (CaO_2) If TL's cardiac output had decreased to 3.5 L/min due to left ventricular injury suffered during his past MI and present STEMI, as well as other factors in his medical/surgical history, what would have been the amount of oxygen delivered to his tissues (D_{O2})? Would TL's D_{O2} have been a cause for concern in this hypothetical situation?

11. TL's body surface area (BSA) was 1.95 m². Calculate his cardiac index if his cardiac output was 3.5 L/min. What is the normal cardiac index range?

12. How are the following oxygenation indices typically affected by a significant decrease in cardiac output?

	NORMAL	INCREASED	DECREASED
$S\bar{v}O_2$			
$P\bar{v}O_2$			
$C\bar{v}O_2$			
$C(a-\bar{v})_{O2}$			
O_2ER			

13. How would severe aortic stenosis affect left ventricular, left atrial, pulmonary venous, and pulmonary capillary pressures? How would it affect the cardiac output and cardiac index?

14. Define myocardial ischemia and myocardial infarction. How can myocardial ischemia and myocardial infarction affect left ventricular contractility?

15. How would a significant decrease in left ventricular contractility affect left ventricular, left atrial, pulmonary venous, and pulmonary capillary pressures? How would it affect the cardiac output and cardiac index?

16. TL's blood pressure remained controlled and relatively stable throughout his ordeal. How does severe hypertension affect left ventricular function? Why was blood pressure control of vital importance to TL?

17. How does IABC therapy assist with cardiac pump function and reduce myocardial ischemia?

18. How does atrial fibrillation, especially atrial fibrillation with a rapid ventricular rate, affect cardiac output? Why was the atrial fibrillation a special concern for TL?

19. Why do patients with chronic atrial fibrillation typically require some kind of anticoagulant medication?

COMMENTS

Over a 36-hour period, TL was weaned from the IABC machine. Over the next four days, TL's condition stabilized to his pre-STEMI status, and he was discharged. The CABG and aortic valve replacement surgery was postponed indefinitely pending TL's decision whether or not to proceed with the surgery.

CASE DISCUSSION

20. If TL had asked for your opinion as to whether or not he should have the surgery, how would you have responded? If you were in TL's position, would you have agreed to the surgery? If you were the physician, how would you have discussed the issue with TL?

CASE STUDY 7

ATELECTASIS

CASE INTRODUCTION

DN presented to the emergency department complaining of right upper quadrant abdominal pain that she had been experiencing for several hours. The pain was accompanied by nausea and vomiting. DN also reported that she had not been feeling very well for the past week. She believed it to be a stomach flu that several family members and friends had experienced over the past month. A CT scan, however, revealed a severely inflamed gall bladder with multiple large gallstones. A diagnosis of acute cholecystitis was determined by the emergency department physician, and DN was admitted to the hospital. Early the next morning, DN underwent laparoscopic cholecystectomy surgery for the removal of her gall bladder. The surgeon's report stated that her gall bladder was gangrenous but had not ruptured. Due to the length of the surgery, as well as DN's age and other health conditions, the decision was made to keep DN intubated and weaned as tolerated from mechanical ventilation. She was transferred to the ICU for further care. DN was intubated with a 7.5 mm endotracheal tube.

INITIAL ASSESSMENT

Age: 80-years-old
Height: 5' 4"
Weight: 140 lbs. (64 kg)
Heart Rate: 108 bpm
Respiratory Rate: 14 bpm
Blood Pressure: 110/70 mm Hg
S_pO_2: 100% (AC 14 500 mL 60% O_2 PEEP +5 cm H_2O)
Temperature: 38.2° C
Breath Sounds: expiratory wheezes (upper lobes), diminished (lower lobes)
Chest/Abdominal Inspection: pectus excavatum
Cough/Sputum: none
Level of Consciousness: obtunded (anesthesia)
Medical/Surgical History: chronic obstructive pulmonary disease (COPD), chronic renal failure (CRF), hypertension, hypothyroidism, appendectomy, cesarean section x 2, hysterectomy
Social History: ex-smoker 1 PPD x 40 years (quit 15 years ago)
Current Medications: albuterol, tiotropium bromide, fluticasone propionate/salmeterol, hydrochlorothiazide, losartan potassium, levothyroxine sodium
Allergies: no known allergies

DIAGNOSTIC RESULTS

Chest X-ray: tip of endotracheal tube 3 cm above carina, mild hyperinflation consistent with COPD

ABG: (AC 14 500 mL 60% O_2 PEEP +5 cm H_2O) (total respiratory rate = 14 bpm)
Hb = 11.0 g/dL
pH = 7.23
$PaCO_2$ = 44 mm Hg
PaO_2 = 176 mm Hg
SaO_2 = 100%
HCO_3^- = 18 mEq/L
BE = $^-$9 mEq/L
CaO_2 = 15.3 Vol%

ABG Interpretation: _____

Complete Blood Count:
White Blood Cells = 10.5 x 10^3/mm^3
Red Blood Cells = 3.92 x 10^6/mm^3
Hemoglobin = 11.4 g/dL
Hematocrit = 35.4%
Platelets = 253 x 10^3/mm^3

Chemistry Profile:
Na^+ = 141 mEq/L
K^+ = 3.8 mEq/L
Cl^- = 113 mEq/L
CO_2 = 19 mEq/L
Glucose = 159 mg/dL
Blood Urea Nitrogen = 33 mg/dL
Creatinine = 1.9 mg/dL
Albumin = 2.8 g/dL
Mg^{2+} = 2.0 mg/dL

Ventilation Mechanics:
Plateau Pressure (P_{PLAT}): 18 cm H_2O
Static Lung Compliance (C_S): 38 mL/cm H_2O
Airway Resistance (R_{AW}): 12 cm H_2O/L/sec

COMMENTS

The ventilator settings were adjusted to: AC 16 500 mL 40% O_2 PEEP +5 cm H_2O.

DIAGNOSTIC RESULTS

ABG: (AC 16 500 mL 40% O_2 PEEP +5 cm H_2O) (total respiratory rate = 16 bpm)

Hb = 10.6 g/dL

pH = 7.32

$PaCO_2$ = 34 mm Hg

PaO_2 = 117 mm Hg

SaO_2 = 100%

HCO_3^- = 17 mEq/L

BE = $^-$8 mEq/L

CaO_2 = 14.6 Vol%

ABG Interpretation: _____

COMMENTS

The ventilator settings were adjusted to: AC 16 500 mL 30% O_2 PEEP +5 cm H_2O.

CASE DISCUSSION

1. Were the initial ventilator settings and subsequent changes appropriate?

2. What does the CO_2 in the chemistry profile measure?

3. Were there any abnormal values in the complete blood count and chemistry profile results?

4. Which factor(s) in the patient assessment likely affected DN's static lung compliance value?

5. What could have been causing the high airway resistance? Are there any recommendations that you would have offered to reduce the airway resistance in this case?

COMMENTS
Over an eight-hour period, DN was successfully weaned from mechanical ventilation and extubated. A post-extubation respiratory therapist assessment was ordered by the ICU intensivist for recommendations.

ASSESSMENT
Heart Rate: 96 bpm
Respiratory Rate: 20 bpm
Blood Pressure: 115/74 mm Hg
S$_p$O$_2$: 88% (room air) 93% (nasal cannula at 2 L/min)
Temperature: 37.5° C
Breath Sounds: expiratory wheezes (upper lobes), diminished (lower lobes)
Chest/Abdominal Inspection: pectus excavatum
Cough/Sputum: fair, guarded, loose, nonproductive
Level of Consciousness: alert/oriented x 3
General Appearance/Behavior: guarding right side, complaining of pain
Medical/Surgical History: chronic obstructive pulmonary disease (COPD), chronic renal failure (CRF), hypertension, hypothyroidsim, appendectomy, cesarean section x 2, hysterectomy
Social History: ex-smoker 1 PPD x 40 years (quit 15 years ago)
Home Respiratory Medications: albuterol 2.5 mg unit dose QID, tiotropium bromide 1 capsule QD (A.M.), fluticasone propionate/salmeterol 250/50 mcg 1 puff BID
Home Oxygen: none
Home CPAP/NPPV: none
Allergies: no known allergies

TREATMENT (RECOMMENDATIONS)
albuterol 2.5 mg unit dose aerosol treatments Q4 hrs while awake + Q2 hrs PRN
tiotropium bromide 1 capsule QD (A.M.)
fluticasone propionate/salmeterol 250/50 mcg 1 puff BID
incentive spirometry 10-15 breaths Q1-2 hrs while awake
O$_2$ via nasal cannula at 2 L/min (titrate to keep S$_p$O$_2$ > 92%)

CASE DISCUSSION
6. How would you describe DN's post-extubation respiratory status?

7. Do you agree with the respiratory therapist's recommendations?

COMMENTS

The intensivist approved the respiratory therapist's recommendations, and treatment was initiated following the administration of morphine sulfate by DN's nurse for pain. DN achieved 1000 mL with the incentive spirometer (1900 mL predicted). Splinting, deep breathing, and coughing instructions were given to DN by the respiratory therapist. While expiratory wheezes were still auscultated, aeration had improved following the albuterol aerosol treatment. DN quickly fell asleep after completion of the respiratory treatments.

At 0300, DN's nurse reported to the respiratory therapist that DN's supplemental oxygen via nasal cannula had been increased to 6 L/min and that her S_pO_2 was only 88%. She also reported that DN's incentive spirometry efforts had decreased to 600 mL. The respiratory therapist exchanged the nasal cannula with a 50% air entrainment mask and completed an assessment.

ASSESSMENT

Heart Rate: 115 bpm
Respiratory Rate: 32 bpm (shallow)
Blood Pressure: 135/84 mm Hg
S_pO_2: 93% (50% air entrainment mask)
Temperature: 38.0° C
Breath Sounds: faint expiratory wheezes (upper lobes), fine crackles (lower lobes), severely diminished throughout all lung fields
Chest/Abdominal Inspection: pectus excavatum, inspiratory and expiratory accessory muscle use
Cough/Sputum: weak, guarded, loose, nonproductive
Level of Consciousness: lethargic
General Appearance/Behavior: lethargic, lying on right side, complaining of pain and dyspnea

COMMENTS

The respiratory therapist obtained an ABG per respiratory protocol and presented her assessment findings along with the ABG results to the intensivist. A chest X-ray was ordered by the intensivist.

DIAGNOSTIC RESULTS

Chest X-ray: right middle and lower lobe consolidation, elevated hemidiaphragm on the right, left lower lobe atelectasis

ABG: (50% air entrainment mask)
Hb = 10.8 g/dL
pH = 7.43
$PaCO_2$ = 28 mm Hg
PaO_2 = 65 mm Hg
SaO_2 = 93%
HCO_3^- = 18 mEq/L
BE = -6 mEq/L
CaO_2 = 13.7 Vol%

ABG Interpretation: _____

CASE DISCUSSION

8. What did the chest X-ray results indicate?

9. What factors led to the development of this respiratory complication?

10. Were any signs observed during the post-extubation assessment indicating that DN's respiratory status was likely to deteriorate during the night?

11. How do you account for the overcompensation in the ABG results?

12. How would you describe DN's oxygenation status?

COMMENTS

The respiratory therapist requested and obtained an order for CPAP. CPAP +8 cm H_2O 50% O_2 was initiated.

CASE DISCUSSION

13. Do you agree with the actions taken by the respiratory therapist?

14. What were the indications for the use of CPAP?

15. Were the CPAP settings appropriate?

COMMENTS

DN used the CPAP until 0800. The oxygen had been weaned down to 35% over the five-hour period. A morning chest X-ray was completed, and DN's scheduled respiratory medications were administered following an assessment.

ASSESSMENT

Heart Rate: 88 bpm
Respiratory Rate: 20 bpm
Blood Pressure: 112/70 mm Hg
S_pO_2: 96% (nasal cannula at 4 L/min)
Temperature: 37.0° C
Breath Sounds: expiratory wheezes (upper lobes), diminished (lower lobes)
Chest/Abdominal Inspection: pectus excavatum
Cough/Sputum: fair, loose, productive/moderate amounts of thin, pale-yellow secretions
Level of Consciousness: alert/oreinted
General Appearance/Behavior: resting comfortably, splinting right side with cough

DIAGNOSTIC RESULTS

Chest X-ray: significant improvement since previous film, atelectasis persists along base of right lower lobe

ABG: (nasal cannula at 4 L/min)

Hb = 10.8 g/dL

pH = 7.37

$PaCO_2$ = 38 mm Hg

PaO_2 = 98 mm Hg

SaO_2 = 97%

HCO_3^- = 21 mEq/L

BE = $^-$3 mEq/L

CaO_2 = 14.3 Vol%

ABG Interpretation: _____

COMMENTS

DN continued to progress well throughout the day. Her nurse had her out of bed and walking or sitting in a chair. She agreed to use the CPAP overnight, and it was discontinued the following morning. She was transferred to a regular medical/surgical unit on room air the same morning. DN's home respiratory medication regimen was resumed, and frequent incentive spirometer use was strongly encouraged. She was discharged two days later.

CASE DISCUSSION

16. List at least five factors that can cause atelectasis due to decreased lung expansion.

17. Explain how airway obstruction and breathing high concentrations of oxygen can lead to atelectasis.

18. How are the following pulmonary function measurements affected by clinically significant atelectasis?

	NORMAL	INCREASED	DECREASED
FVC			
FEV$_1$			
FEV$_{1\%}$			
IRV			
V$_T$			
IC			
ERV			
VC			
RV			
FRC			
TLC			
RV/TLC RATIO			

19. What chest palpation and percussion assessment findings are associated with atelectasis?

20. Which lung volume or capacity does incentive spirometry measure?

21. In addition to CPAP, what other respiratory care interventions are helpful in the reversal of atelectasis?

22. List at least three extrapulmonary causes of lung compression atelectasis.

23. To which side does the mediastinum shift in a severe case of atelectasis?

24. Was the CPAP indicated for the second night of DN's stay in the ICU?

CASE STUDY 8

CHRONIC BRONCHITIS/EMPHYSEMA (COPD)

CASE INTRODUCTION

HG was transported to the hospital by her husband following two days of increasing shortness of breath. She stated that she was reluctant to return to the hospital because she had just been discharged two weeks earlier after a seven-day admission for a COPD exacerbation. The hospital staff was accustomed to caring for HG since the frequency of her hospital admissions had been increasing over the past two years. She was lightheartedly referred to as a "frequent flyer" by the respiratory care staff which bonded with her and her family over the years.

INITIAL ASSESSMENT

Age: 65-years-old
Height: 5' 6"
Weight: 120 lbs. (55 kg)
Heart Rate: 120 bpm
Respiratory Rate: 32 bpm
Blood Pressure: 156/90 mm Hg
S$_p$O$_2$: 87% (nasal cannula at 3 L/min)
Temperature: 38.5° C
Breath Sounds: severely diminished throughout all lung fields
Chest/Abdominal Inspection: expiratory accessory muscle use, abdominal paradox, increased anterior-posterior diameter
Cough/Sputum: weak, congested, productive/large amounts of thick, yellow sputum
Level of Consciousness: alert/oriented x 3
General Appearance/Behavior: cachectic, anxious, pursed-lip breathing, tripod position
Medical/Surgical History: chronic obstructive pulmonary disease (COPD), hypertension, atrial fibrillation, hernia repair
Social History: ex-smoker 1-2 PPD x 45 years (quit 1 year ago)
Current Medications: albuterol, fluticasone propionate/salmeterol, tiotropium bromide, prednisone, warfarin sodium, diltiazem
Allergies: penicillin

DIAGNOSTIC RESULTS
ABG: (nasal cannula at 3 L/min)

Hb = 13.2 g/dL

pH = 7.28

$PaCO_2$ = 63 mm Hg

PaO_2 = 54 mm Hg

SaO_2 = 87%

HCO_3^- = 29 mEq/L

BE = 2 mEq/L

CaO_2 = 15.6 Vol%

ABG Interpretation: _____

INITIAL TREATMENT
albuterol 2.5 mg unit dose aerosol treatment x 3

methylprednisolone 125 mg IV

levofloxacin 750 mg IV

aztreonam 2g IV

lorazepam 1 mg IV

normal saline IV fluids at 100 mL/hr

bi-level NPPV (noninvasive positive pressure ventilation) 14 cm H_2O/6 cm H_2O 40% O_2 (titrate O_2 to keep S_pO_2 > 92%)

DIAGNOSTIC RESULTS
Chest X-ray: severe COPD, right hilar infiltrate

Complete Blood Count:

White Blood Cells = 21.1 x 10^3/mm^3

Red Blood Cells = 4.07 x 10^6/mm^3

Hemoglobin = 13.2 g/dL

Hematocrit = 38.5%

Platelets = 274 x 10^3/mm^3

Chemistry Profile:

Na^+ = 138 mEq/L

K^+ = 4.6mEq/L

Cl^- = 100 mEq/L

CO_2 = 29 mEq/L

Glucose = 103 mg/dL

Blood Urea Nitrogen = 31 mg/dL

Creatinine = 0.6 mg/dL

Albumin = 3.1 g/dL

Mg^{2+} = 1.8 mg/dL

TREATMENT
magnesium sulfate 2g IV

COMMENTS

HG expectorated large amounts of thick, yellow secretions following the three aerosol treatments. A sputum sample was sent to the laboratory for analysis. Her breath sounds remained severely diminished throughout all lung fields. Faint expiratory wheezes were auscultated in the upper lung regions. HG tolerated the bi-level NPPV therapy well. Exhaled tidal volumes ranged between 400 and 450 mL, and her total respiratory rate remained between 12 and 16 bpm. She was admitted to the ICU for a COPD exacerbation and pneumonia.

CASE DISCUSSION

1. Calculate HG's ideal body weight (IBW). If HG required mechanical ventilation, which weight would you use to determine her set tidal volume for mandatory breaths?

2. List at least three assessment and/or diagnostic findings to support the diagnosis of pneumonia.

3. What are the physiologic effects of bi-level NPPV?

4. Were the bi-level NPPV settings appropriate?

5. What was one potential drawback to the use of bi-level NPPV in this case?

6. Would CPAP have been a viable alternative to bi-level NPPV?

7. What radiologic findings would be consistent with a "severe COPD" interpretation for HG's chest X-ray?

8. Why is the administration of magnesium sulfate helpful for patients with an increased work of breathing?

9. Explain the physiologic effects of pursed-lip breathing.

10. What was the primary reason for the administration of lorazepam in this case?

11. What potential deleterious effect(s) could result from the use of lorazepam or other anti-anxiety medications for patients in respiratory distress?

DIAGNOSTIC RESULTS
ABG: (bi-level NPPV 14 cm H_2O/6 cm H_2O 40% O_2-two hours after bi-level NPPV initiated)
Hb = 13.0 g/dL
pH = 7.35
$PaCO_2$ = 45 mm Hg
PaO_2 = 70 mm Hg
SaO_2 = 93%
HCO_3^- = 24 mEq/L
BE = $^-$1 mEq/L
CaO_2 = 15.3 Vol%

ABG Interpretation: _____

COMMENTS
Upon arrival in the ICU, the ICU intensivist ordered a respiratory therapist evaluation for recommendations.

ASSESSMENT
Heart Rate: 110 bpm
Respiratory Rate: 20 bpm
Blood Pressure: 128/84 mm Hg
S_pO_2: 93% (bi-level NPPV 14 cm H_2O/6 cm H_2O 40% O_2)
Temperature: 37.8° C
Breath Sounds: faint expiratory wheezes (upper lobes), severely diminished throughout all lung fields
Chest/Abdominal Inspection: increased anterior-posterior diameter
Cough/Sputum: none
Level of Consciousness: alert/oriented x 3
General Appearance/Behavior: cachectic, resting comfortably
Medical/Surgical History: COPD, hypertension, atrial fibrillation, hernia repair
Social History: ex-smoker 1-2 PPD x 45 years (quit 1 year ago)
Current Respiratory Medications: albuterol 2.5 mg unit dose aerosol treatments 4-5 times per day, albuterol MDI PRN, fluticasone propionate/salmeterol 250/50 mcg 1 puff BID, tiotropium bromide 1 capsule QD, prednisone10 mg QD
Home Oxygen: nasal cannula at 3 L/min (continuously)
Home CPAP/NPPV: none
Allergies: penicillin

TREATMENT (RECOMMENDATIONS)

albuterol 2.5 mg unit dose aerosol treatments Q4 hrs while awake + Q2 hrs PRN tiotropium bromide 1 capsule QD (A.M.) fluticasone propionate/salmeterol 250/50 mcg 1 puff BID PEP (positive expiratory pressure) therapy with aerosol treatments

O_2 via nasal cannula at 3 L/min (titrate to keep $S_pO_2 > 92\%$) bi-level NPPV 14 cm H_2O/6 cm H_2O 40% O_2 while sleeping and as needed

COMMENTS

The intensivist agreed with the respiratory therapist's recommendations, and treatment continued as recommended. HG was transferred to a medical/surgical unit on the third day of her hospital stay. The aztreonam was discontinued on the second day after Streptococcal pneumoniae was identified as the source of the pneumonia. The levofloxacin was continued throughout HG's seven-day hospital stay. The methylprednisolone was weaned down and discontinued over the same period, and HG's home regimen of prednisone was resumed. HG continued to use bi-level NPPV at night, and the process for acquiring bi-level NPPV for home use was completed. A nasal mask was used during the last three nights to which HG adapted without any difficulty. A respiratory therapist completed an assessment the morning HG was discharged from the hospital.

ASSESSMENT

Heart Rate: 104 bpm
Respiratory Rate: 24 bpm
Blood Pressure: 118/76 mm Hg
S_pO_2: 93% (nasal cannula at 3 L/min)
Temperature: 37.0° C
Breath Sounds: clear (upper lobes), diminished throughout all lung fields
Chest/Abdominal Inspection: mild expiratory accessory muscle use, increased anterior-posterior diameter
Cough/Sputum: fair, loose, nonproductive
Level of Consciousness: alert/oriented x 3
General Appearance/Behavior: cachectic, pursed-lip breathing, resting comfortably, excited about being discharged

CASE DISCUSSION

12. Do you agree with the respiratory care plan that was implemented for HG?

13. What are some specific respiratory care interventions that provide PEP therapy?

14. Which of the assessment findings were chronic and persisted after HG was discharged?

15. Why was HG an ideal candidate for nocturnal bi-level NPPV?

16. Compare and contrast the physiologic or structural changes associated with chronic bronchitis and emphysema.

CHRONIC BRONCHITIS	EMPHYSEMA

17. How are the pathologic or structural changes associated with chronic bronchitis and emphysema typically addressed in a respiratory care plan?

18. What is the difference between panlobular emphysema and centrilobular emphysema?

19. How does alpha$_1$-antitrypsin protect the lungs?

20. List at least four etiological factors that are known to cause chronic bronchitis or emphysema.

21. Why are patients with chronic bronchitis or emphysema more likely to develop respiratory infections?

22. What chest palpation and percussion assessment findings are associated with COPD-related hyperinflation?

23. How would you identify an acute alveolar hyperventilation superimposed on a chronic ventilatory failure when analyzing ABG results?

24. How would you identify an acute ventilatory failure superimposed on a chronic ventilatory failure when analyzing ABG results?

25. How are the following hemodynamic indices typically affected by chronic bronchitis and emphysema?

	NORMAL	INCREASED	DECREASED
PVR			
PAP			
CVP			
RVSWI			
PCWP			
SVR			
CO			
CI			
LVSWI			

26. How does cor pulmonale develop?

27. How are the following pulmonary function measurements typically affected by chronic bronchitis and emphysema?

	NORMAL	INCREASED	DECREASED
FVC			
FEV_1			
$FEV_{1\%}$			
PEFR			
RV			
ERV			
FRC			
TLC			
RV/TLC RATIO			

28. Why does breathing moderate to high concentrations of oxygen cause some COPD patients with chronic hypercapnia to hypoventilate?

Reference:

Wilkins, R.L., Stoller, J.K., & Kacmarek, R.M. (2009). *Egan's fundamentals of respiratory care* (9th ed.). St. Louis: Mosby (pp. 309-313).

29. The respiratory care staff had an ideal working relationship with HG and her family. How would you cope with the frequent flyer patient who might not be as friendly or cooperative as HG?

CASE STUDY 9

ASPIRATION PNEUMONIA

CASE INTRODUCTION

GW was found around midnight in his dormitory room in a pool of vomit by his roommate. GW had been to a fraternity party earlier in the evening and had engaged in heavy alcohol consumption. GW's roommate rolled GW over onto his side and called EMS. EMS personnel arrived to find GW unresponsive and agonal breathing. They successfully intubated GW with an 8.0 mm endotracheal tube on the first attempt and suctioned the endotracheal tube several times. Copious amounts of fluid and partially digested food were suctioned. GW was manually ventilated with 100% oxygen via a bag-valve resuscitator during the transport to the local emergency department.

INITIAL ASSESSMENT

Age: 22-years-old
Height: 6' 3"
Weight: 200 lbs. (91 kg)
Heart Rate: 56 bpm
Respiratory Rate: 12 bpm (manual ventilation with bag-valve resuscitator)
Blood Pressure: 100/60 mm Hg
S$_p$O$_2$: 98% (100% O$_2$ via bag-valve resuscitator)
Temperature: 36.5° C
Breath Sounds: absent (right lung), wheezes and rhonchi (left upper lobe), diminished (left lower lobe)
Chest/Abdominal Inspection: significantly decreased chest expansion on right side
Cough/Sputum: suctioning required/small amounts of fluid and partially digested food
Level of Consciousness: comatose
Medical/Surgical History: unknown
Social History: unknown
Current Medications: unknown
Allergies: unknown
(NOTE: GW's parents had been notified and were en route to the hospital.)

COMMENTS

GW developed ventricular fibrillation shortly after arriving at the emergency department and was defibrillated twice in order to return his heart rhythm to normal sinus at a rate of 64 bpm. An ABG was drawn, and a bronchoscopy was emergently performed.

DIAGNOSTIC RESULTS

ABG: (100% O_2 via bag-valve resuscitator)

Hb = 11.5 g/dL

pH = 7.10

$PaCO_2$ = 55 mm Hg

PaO_2 = 125 mm Hg

SaO_2 = 100%

HCO_3^- = 17 mEq/L

BE = $^-$11 mEq/L

CaO_2 = 15.8 Vol%

ABG Interpretation: _____

BRONCHOSCOPY REPORT

A large food bolus was removed from the distal end of the right mainstem bronchus. Other food substances were removed from the lobar bronchi of both lungs. All of the proximal airways (trachea, mainstem bronchi, and lobar bronchi) showed signs of severe inflammation.

COMMENTS

Breath sounds improved over both lungs following the bronchoscopy. Mechanical ventilation was initiated. Initial ventilator settings were: PC/AC 20/14 60% O_2 PEEP +10 cm H_2O T_I = 1.0 sec (titrate to keep exhaled tidal volume 500-550 mL). GW's parents arrived at the emergency department and provided the missing assessment information.

INITIAL ASSESSMENT (ADDENDUM)

Medical/Surgical History: severe concussion with post-concussion seizures (football injury six years ago)

Social History: non-smoker

Current Medications: phenytoin

Allergies: no known allergies

DIAGNOSTIC RESULTS

Chest X-ray: (after bronchoscopy) tip of endotracheal tube 2.5 cm above carina, multiple patchy infiltrates throughout both lungs, atelectatic changes in right lower lobe

ETOH: 0.321 g/dL

phenytoin: 6 mcg/mL (10-20 mcg/mL therapeutic range)

ABG: (PC/AC 20/14 60% O_2 PEEP +10 cm H_2O T_I = 1.0 sec) (exhaled tidal volume = 550 mL, total respiratory rate = 14 bpm)

Hb = 10.5 g/dL

pH = 7.37

$PaCO_2$ = 35 mm Hg

PaO_2 = 155 mm Hg

SaO_2 = 100%

HCO_3^- = 20 mEq/L

BE = $^-$5 mEq/L

CaO_2 = 14.5 Vol%

ABG Interpretation: _____

COMMENTS

Ventilator settings were adjusted to: PC/AC 20/14 40% O_2 PEEP +10 cm H_2O T_I = 1.0 sec.

CASE DISCUSSION

1. Based on the available information at this point in the case study, what do you suspect caused GW's current condition?

2. Why would you have expected a metabolic acidosis component in the ABG results in this case?

3. Why do you think pressure control ventilation was chosen over volume ventilation?

4. Were the initial ventilator settings and subsequent changes appropriate?

COMMENTS

GW was transferred to the ICU. A radial arterial catheter and pulmonary artery catheter were inserted by the ICU intensivist. Fluid resuscitation to correct the metabolic acidosis that was initiated in the emergency department was continued. Over the next eight hours, GW's condition stabilized. GW's level of consciousness improved, and he responded to commands. He became increasingly agitated, and a propofol drip was started to maintain adequate sedation.

DIAGNOSTIC RESULTS

ABG: (PC/AC 20/14 40% O_2 PEEP +10 cm H_2O T_I = 1.0 sec) (exhaled tidal volume = 550 mL, total respiratory rate = 14 bpm)

Hb = 10.0 g/dL

pH = 7.42

$PaCO_2$ = 37 mm Hg

PaO_2 = 88 mm Hg

SaO_2 = 96%

HCO_3^- = 23 mEq/L

BE = $^-$1 mEq/L

CaO_2 = 13.1 Vol%

ABG Interpretation: _____

Urine Output: 40 mL/hr

CASE DISCUSSION

5. How would you describe GW's oxygenation status?

6. What is considered a normal urine output? What is the minimum mean arterial pressure required to maintain kidney function?

7. Which hemodynamic measurement(s) would you have used to monitor GW's fluid status? Why would the monitoring of GW's fluid status have been of vital importance in this case?

COMMENTS

During the night, a respiratory therapist noticed that the exhaled tidal volume had decreased to 450 mL and the S_pO_2 had decreased to 91%. GW was appropriately sedated, and the total respiratory rate was 14 bpm. No change in tidal volume was observed after suctioning.

CASE DISCUSSION

8. What do you suspect caused the observed changes?

DIAGNOSTIC RESULTS

ABG: (PC/AC 20/14 40% O_2 PEEP +10 cm H_2O T_I = 1.0 sec) (exhaled tidal volume = 450 mL, total respiratory rate = 14 bpm)

Hb = 10.2 g/dL
pH = 7.25
$PaCO_2$ = 53 mm Hg
PaO_2 = 61 mm Hg
SaO_2 = 91%
HCO_3^- = 22 mEq/L
BE = $^-$4 mEq/L
CaO_2 = 12.6 Vol%

ABG Interpretation: _____

CASE DISCUSSION

9. How would you describe GW's oxygenation status?

10. Calculate the change in static lung compliance that occurred since mechanical ventilation was initiated.

11. The respiratory rate was increased to 20 bpm which corrected the respiratory component of the acidosis. What ventilator setting adjustment was necessary to increase the I:E ratio to 1:1 as requested by the intensivist?

12. If GW's exhaled tidal volume continued to decrease, what would you have recommended?

13. What assessment findings or diagnostic results would have indicated that GW was ready to be weaned?

14. How would you have proceeded to wean GW if the respiratory rate was 20 bpm, the pressure was 20 cm H_2O, and the I:E ratio was 1:1?

COMMENTS

By the eighth day of GW's ICU admission, he had been weaned to CPAP +8 cm H_2O 30% O_2 PS +15 cm H_2O. He underwent a tracheotomy procedure on the ninth day and was transferred to a long-term acute care facility on the twelfth day. At the time GW was transferred, the prognosis for a full recovery was good, but the possibility of neurological and/or neuromuscular deficits did exist considering the anoxic brain injury GW suffered.

15. What might future pulmonary function test results reveal about GW's lung function?

16. What kind of bacterial infections are associated with the aspiration of gastric contents?

17. What is meant by the term "aspiration pneumonitis"?

18. How does the pH of aspirated gastric contents affect the degree of lung injury?

19. Why is acute respiratory distress syndrome (ARDS) frequently associated with aspiration pneumonia?

CASE STUDY 10

PULMONARY EMBOLISM

CASE INTRODUCTION

SV was transported to the emergency department by EMS personnel after developing severe pain in her right upper back and shortness of breath. She had been discharged from the hospital the previous day following a four-day admission for symptomatic bradycardia. SV had a pacemaker inserted during her hospital stay.

INITIAL ASSESSMENT

Age: 70-years-old
Height: 5' 8"
Weight: 172 lbs. (78 kg)
Heart Rate: 118 bpm
Respiratory Rate: 32 bpm
Blood Pressure: 158/90 mm Hg
S$_p$O$_2$: 89% (room air)
Temperature: 37.0° C
Breath Sounds: clear (upper lobes), crackles (lower lobes), diminished throughout all lung fields
Chest/Abdominal Inspection: decreased chest expansion (decreased inspiratory efforts due to severe back pain)
Cough/Sputum: fair, loose, productive/small amounts of blood-tinged sputum
Level of Consciousness: alert/oriented x 3
General Appearance/Behavior: anxious, complaining of right upper back pain
Medical/Surgical History: hypertension, bradycardia, pacemaker insertion, kidney stones, lithotripsy, arthroscopic surgery on right knee, thrombectomy right leg
Social History: non-smoker
Current Medications: lisinopril, amlodipine
Allergies: meperidine hydrochloride

DIAGNOSTIC RESULTS

ECG: sinus tachycardia

Chest X-ray: mild cardiomegaly, area of increased density within right lower lobe may represent infiltrate or atelectasis

Chest CT: multiple acute pulmonary emboli within right pulmonary artery branches

ABG: (room air) (P_B = 750 mm Hg)

Hb = 15.8 g/dL

pH = 7.58

$PaCO_2$ = 20 mm Hg

PaO_2 = 57 mm Hg

SaO_2 = 88%

HCO_3^- = 18 mEq/L

BE = $^-$4 mEq/L

CaO_2 = 18.8 Vol%

ABG Interpretation: _____

Complete Blood Count:

White Blood Cells = 8.2 x 10^3/mm^3

Red Blood Cells = 5.22 x 10^6/mm^3

Hemoglobin = 15.7 g/dL

Hematocrit = 46.2%

Platelets = 211 x 10^3/mm^3

Chemistry Profile:

Na^+ = 138 mEq/L

K^+ = 4.1 mEq/L

Cl^- = 105 mEq/L

CO_2 = 21 mEq/L

Glucose = 136 mg/dL

Blood Urea Nitrogen = 19 mg/dL

Creatinine = 1.0 mg/dL

Albumin = 4.4 g/dL

Mg^{2+} = 2.0 mg/dL

Cardiac Profile:

Creatine Kinase: 114 U/L

Creatine Kinase-MB: 1.5 ng/mL

Troponin: 0.02 ng/mL

B-type Natriuretic Peptide (BNP): 25 pg/mL

Coagulation Profile:

International Normalized Ratio (INR): 1.11

Prothrombin Time (PT): 11.8 sec

Activated Partial Thromboplastin Time (PTT): 28.1 sec

INITIAL TREATMENT
50% air entrainment mask
heparin 6240 U IV bolus (80 U/kg)
heparin drip IV (per protocol)
morphine sulfate 2 mg IV

COMMENTS
SV was admitted to the ICU. The heparin drip per pulmonary embolism protocol was continued. Over the next eight hours, SV's S_pO_2 increased to 93% on the 50% air entrainment mask, and her respiratory rate decreased to 28 bpm. SV continued to complain of pain in her right upper back, but the subjective pain level had decreased from a rating of 10 to a rating of 4. SV's blood pressure decreased to 124/82 mm Hg and remained stable throughout her entire five-day hospital admission.

DIAGNOSTIC RESULTS
Venous Duplex Scan: (bilateral legs) negative for deep venous thrombosis

CASE DISCUSSION
1. Calculate SV's alveolar-arterial oxygen gradient $(P(A-a)_{O_2})$. What is the normal $P(A-a)_{O_2}$ range on room air? Is the calculation of the $P(A-a)_{O_2}$ useful in a suspected pulmonary embolism situation?

2. A patient who is hyperventilating secondary to anxiety may have a clinical presentation similar to a patient with a pulmonary embolism. Assuming an anxious patient is free of pulmonary disease, what would you expect the $P(A-a)_{O_2}$ calculation to show?

3. What would the ABG results likely reveal for an extensive pulmonary embolism with infarction?

4. Which of SV's assessment findings are typically associated with a pulmonary embolism? Are any of these assessment findings specific for a pulmonary embolism?

5. A D-dimer test is often obtained for a patient experiencing chest pain. What does the D-dimer test measure? How are the results of the D-dimer test used? Why do you suppose the D-dimer test was not ordered for SV?

6. Except for the ABG results, were there any clues in any of the laboratory results to indicate an increased probability of a pulmonary embolism?

7. How does the blood-tinged sputum that is often associated with a pulmonary embolism develop?

8. What are the three major mechanisms causing pulmonary hypertension as the result of a pulmonary embolism?

9. How can severe pulmonary hypertension affect the systemic blood pressure?

10. How would a pulmonary embolism likely affect the following hemodynamic indices?

	NORMAL	INCREASED	DECREASED
PVR			
PAP			
CVP			
RVSWI			

11. How would an extensive pulmonary embolism likely affect the following hemodynamic indices?

	NORMAL	INCREASED	DECREASED
PCWP			
SV			
CO			
CI			
SVR			
LVSWI			

12. How does a pulmonary embolism initially affect the ventilation/perfusion ratio?

13. What pathologic or structural changes can cause a decrease in the ventilation/perfusion ratio when a pulmonary embolism is present?

14. How is the dead space/tidal volume (V_D/V_T) ratio calculated for a patient being mechanically ventilated? What is the normal V_D/V_T ratio?

15. What are the hazards of using high concentrations of oxygen for a patient with a pulmonary embolism?

16. What causes the bronchospasm occasionally associated with a pulmonary embolism? How can bronchospasm worsen pulmonary vasoconstriction?

17. What chest X-ray findings might be present if lung tissue is infarcted due to a pulmonary embolism? What is Westermark's sign?

18. How is a ventilation/perfusion scan used to identify a pulmonary embolism?

19. What is a saddle embolism? What prognosis is generally associated with a saddle embolism?

COMMENTS

SV responded exceptionally well to the heparin therapy. By the third day, she was on room air, asymptomatic, and anxious to return home. A warfarin regimen was started on the fourth day which was to be continued after discharge. Following a patient education session involving SV and her husband regarding warfarin therapy, SV was discharged late on the fifth day of her hospital admission.

CASE STUDY 11

CHEST TRAUMA

CASE INTRODUCTION

RS was driving home from work around midnight when he was hit by another car failing to stop at a traffic light. The primary impact was on the driver's side door at approximately 45 miles per hour. Fire department personnel arrived on the scene within ten minutes and quickly extricated RS from his vehicle. EMS personnel transported RS to a local emergency department to be stabilized before being transported to the regional trauma center. Due to severe thunderstorms with heavy rains occurring throughout the area, helicopter transport to the trauma center 28 miles away from the receiving hospital was not an option.

INITIAL ASSESSMENT

Age: 30-years-old
Height: 6' 2"
Weight: 175 lbs. (80 kg)
Heart Rate: 68 bpm
Respiratory Rate: 32 bpm
Blood Pressure: 128/82 mm Hg
S$_p$O$_2$: 87% (non-rebreathing mask at 15 L/min)
Temperature: 36.4° C
Breath Sounds: severely diminished (left lung), clear (right upper lobe), diminished (right lower lobes)
Chest/Abdominal Inspection: paradoxical movement of left chest wall
Cough/Sputum: weak, congested, productive/small amounts of bright red blood-tinged sputum
Level of Consciousness: confused
General Appearance/Behavior: air splint on left arm, thick dressing secured on left side of head, cervical collar properly positioned, secured on backboard, severely agitated
Medical/Surgical History: unknown
Social History: unknown
Current Medications: unknown
Allergies: unknown

COMMENTS

RS was immediately intubated with a 7.5 mm endotracheal tube following the administration of etomidate and rocuronium. A fiberoptic bronchoscope was used for the intubation due to the potential degree of difficulty posed by the cervical collar and backboard. Initial ventilator settings were: AC 10 500 mL 60% O$_2$ PEEP +8 cm H$_2$O. A fentanyl drip was started to maintain sedation. A radial arterial catheter and a central venous catheter were inserted.

DIAGNOSTIC RESULTS

Chest X-ray: tip of endotracheal tube 3.5 cm above carina, increased opacity throughout left lung, right lung well-aerated and clear, multiple fractures of left ribs five through ten, elevated left hemidiaphragm, non-displaced fracture of left clavicle, multiple fractures of left humerus

ABG: (AC 10 500 mL 60% O_2 PEEP +8 cm H_2O) (total respiratory rate = 10 bpm)
Hb = 11.2 g/dL
pH = 7.25
$PaCO_2$ = 50 mm Hg
PaO_2 = 96 mm Hg
SaO_2 = 98%
HCO_3^- = 21 mEq/L
BE = $^-$5 mEq/L
CaO_2 = 15.0 Vol%

ABG Interpretation: _____

COMMENTS

Ventilator settings were adjusted to: AC 14 500 mL 60% O_2 PEEP +8 cm H_2O following the ABG.

DIAGNOSTIC RESULTS

Head CT: negative

Neck CT: negative

Chest CT: significant atelectasis throughout left lung, multiple fractures of left ribs five through ten, left hemidiaphragm elevation, non-displaced fracture of left clavicle

Abdomen CT: negative

Pelvis CT: negative

ABG: (AC 14 500 mL 60% O_2 PEEP +8 cm H_2O) (total respiratory rate = 14 bpm)
Hb = 10.7 g/dL
pH = 7.35
$PaCO_2$ = 43 mm Hg
PaO_2 = 120 mm Hg
SaO_2 = 100%
HCO_3^- = 23 mEq/L
BE = $^-$2 mEq/L
CaO_2 = 14.7 Vol%

ABG Interpretation: _____

COMMENTS

Ventilator settings were adjusted to: AC 14 500 mL 50% O_2 PEEP +8 cm H_2O.

CASE DISCUSSION

1. What type of pulmonary condition did RS have based on the initial assessment findings and diagnostic results?

2. What causes the paradoxical chest wall movement that is sometimes associated with chest trauma?

3. Describe the pendelluft effect.

4. How do the pendelluft effect, lung compression, and atelectasis affect the ventilation/perfusion ratio?

5. Which of RS's assessment findings are consistent with a lung contusion?

6. List the indication(s) for mechanical ventilation in this case.

7. Were the initial ventilator settings and subsequent changes appropriate?

8. Why do you suppose fentanyl was used for sedation rather than propofol?

COMMENTS

Approximately 30 minutes after mechanical ventilation was initiated, RS's blood pressure suddenly decreased to 70/50 mm Hg, his heart rate decreased to 30 bpm, the peak inspiratory pressure was 50 cm H_2O, the exhaled tidal volumes were less than 50 mL per breath, and RS's S_pO_2 had decreased to 68%.

CASE DISCUSSION

9. What do you suppose caused the sudden deterioration in RS's cardiopulmonary status? What is the emergent treatment for this life-threatening complication?

10. What was the likely cause for the significant decrease in RS's blood pressure? How is the pulse pressure calculated? What is the significance of a decreased pulse pressure?

11. What breath sounds would you have expected to auscultate over RS's left lung?

12. What happens to the visceral and parietal pleura when a pneumothorax exists? What happens to the underlying lung?

13. What is the difference between an open and closed pneumothorax?

14. Under what conditions can a penetrating chest wound result in a closed pneumothorax?

15. To which side does the trachea shift when a pneumothorax is present?

16. How is a pneumothorax identified on a chest X-ray?

17. What is the standard treatment for a significant pneumothorax?

18. What are air cysts, blebs, and bullae? Why are they a concern when identified on a chest X-ray or chest CT?

19. List at least three causes of an iatrogenic pneumothorax.

20. Describe how a pleurodesis procedure is performed. What is the goal of a pleurodesis procedure?

COMMENTS

RS was transported by ground to the regional trauma center within two hours of his admission to the emergency department. He underwent a five-hour operation later in the evening to repair his fractured humerus. Extubation was delayed when a left lower lobe pneumonia developed on the seventh day. He received mechanical ventilation for a total of 10 days. He was discharged six days after extubation and was expected to make a full recovery.

CASE STUDY 12

PEDIATRIC PNEUMONIA

CASE INTRODUCTION

The parents of PT thought it was odd that their 4-year-old son had not been up and around early one morning as he usually was. When they checked on him, they found him difficult to arouse, febrile, and tachypneic. They immediately transported him to the local emergency department which was located just a few minutes away from their home.

INITIAL ASSESSMENT

Age: 4-years-old
Weight: 37 lbs. (17 kg)
Heart Rate: 132 bpm
Respiratory Rate: 60 bpm (shallow)
Blood Pressure: 82/44 mm Hg
S$_p$O$_2$: 88% (room air)
Temperature: 39.2° C
Breath Sounds: clear (right lung), diminished (left upper lobe), absent (left lower lobe)
Chest/Abdominal Inspection: decreased chest expansion on left, abdominal paradox
Cough/Sputum: none
Level of Consciousness: obtunded
General Appearance/Behavior: pale, dry, dark and sunken eyes, listless
Medical/Surgical History: none
Current Medications: none
Allergies: no known allergies

INITIAL TREATMENT

340 mL normal saline IV bolus x 2
ceftriaxone sodium 1g IV
azithromycin 300 mg PO
acetaminophen 240 mg PO
ibuprofen 85 mg PO
albuterol/ipratropium bromide unit dose aerosol treatment x 1
albuterol 2.5 mg unit dose aerosol treatment x 2
oxygen via nasal cannula at 2 L/min (titrate to keep S$_p$O$_2$ > 94%)

DIAGNOSTIC RESULTS

Chest X-ray: infiltrate left upper lobe, consolidation left lower lobe, small infiltrate right upper lobe, elevated left hemidiaphragm

CASE DISCUSSION

1. Which of the assessment findings were at least partially affected by dehydration?

2. List at least three factors that would have caused an increased respiratory rate in this case?

3. Explain how the abdominal paradoxical breathing pattern develops?

4. What chest palpation and percussion assessment findings would you have expected over PT's left lower lobe?

5. What were the indications for the bronchodilator aerosol treatments?

COMMENTS

Intravenous access was obtained on the fifth attempt by the emergency department nurses and physicians. PT responded well to the fluid boluses once intravenous access was established. Within 30 minutes, he was alert and resting comfortably. PT's parents stated that he had been at a cousin's birthday party three days earlier, and all of the other children at the party seemed to be healthy. They were surprised that PT could get that sick over a 10-hour period. Although PT had an occasional runny nose during the day, he had no other signs or complaints of being sick at his regular bedtime.

ASSESSMENT
(1 hour after initiation of treatment)
Heart Rate: 120 bpm
Respiratory Rate: 44 bpm
Blood Pressure: 96/58 mm Hg
S_pO_2: 96% (nasal cannula at 3 L/min)
Temperature: 38.0° C
Breath Sounds: wheezes/rhonchi (right upper lobe), clear (right lower lobe), wheezes/rhonchi (left upper lobe), crackles/diminished (left lower lobe)
Chest/Abdominal Inspection: improved chest expansion on left, abdominal paradox
Cough/Sputum: fair, congested, nonproductive
Level of Consciousness: alert
General Appearance/Behavior: pale, dry, dark and sunken eyes, quiet, resting comfortably

DIAGNOSTIC RESULTS
Complete Blood Count:
White Blood Cells = 14.8 x 10^3/mm^3
Red Blood Cells = 4.75 x 10^6/mm^3
Hemoglobin = 13.5 g/dL
Hematocrit = 40.5%
Platelets = 275 x 10^3/mm^3

Chemistry Profile:
Na^+ = 136 mEq/L
K^+ = 3.9 mEq/L
Cl^- = 103 mEq/L
CO_2 = 19 mEq/L
Glucose = 101 mg/dL
Blood Urea Nitrogen = 13 mg/dL
Creatinine = 0.4 mg/dL
Mg^{2+} = 2.3 mg/dL

CASE DISCUSSION
6. What was the significance of the multiple attempts to establish intravenous access for PT?

GARY A. KORZAN MS RRT

7. List at least five assessment findings indicating that PT had a positive response to the fluid boluses.

8. What typically happens to inspissated secretions as they become hydrated? What problems can the hydration of inspissated secretions cause? How should these problems be addressed in a respiratory care plan?

9. Which assessment findings support the premise that the inspissated secretions had been hydrated and were more mobile in this case?

10. Formulate an initial respiratory care plan that could have been used for PT on admission to the pediatric unit.

COMMENTS

PT received aggressive respiratory care during his admission, and he made steady progress. He was discharged on the morning of the fifth day. PT's parents received instructions on postural drainage and chest percussion for the left lower lobe which was to be performed three times a day while completing the 10-day course of antibiotics. Arrangements for a home nebulizer were also completed so aerosol treatments could be administered prior to the bronchial hygiene sessions. PT's pediatrician extended the entire home care plan an additional four days when a chest X-ray taken during a follow-up appointment on the eleventh day revealed a small, persistent infiltrate in PT's left lower lobe.

ASSESSMENT

(Prior to discharge)

Heart Rate: 96 bpm

Respiratory Rate: 24 bpm

Blood Pressure: 94/52 mm Hg

S_pO_2: 98% (room air)

Temperature: 37.2° C

Breath Sounds: clear (right lung), end-expiratory wheezes (left upper lobe), coarse crackles (left lower lobe)

Chest/Abdominal Inspection: normal

Cough/Sputum: fair, loose, productive/small amounts of pale yellow sputum

Level of Consciousness: alert

General Appearance/Behavior: normal, anxious to go home

CASE DISCUSSION

11. Do you agree with the physician's decision to discharge PT?

12. How would you have instructed PT's parents to perform the postural drainage and chest percussion for PT's left lower lobe?

13. What are some of the hazards and complications of postural drainage and chest percussion that you would have discussed with PT's parents?

14. List the physiologic or structural changes associated with pneumonia.

15. List at least three specific causes of the hypoxemia that is often associated with pneumonia.

16. List some of the symptoms or signs that would typically present prior to the development of pneumonia in the pediatric population?

17. What is the purpose of nasal flaring often displayed by infants and children experiencing respiratory distress?

18. What is the purpose of expiratory grunting often displayed by infants and children experiencing respiratory distress?

19. What role does secondhand cigarette smoke play in the development of pneumonia?

20. PT was cooperative with all of the respiratory therapy he received. What strategies would you use to administer respiratory therapy to uncooperative pediatric patients?

CASE STUDY 13

NEAR DROWNING

CASE INTRODUCTION

LE was swimming at a northern Ohio public beach along Lake Erie on a mid-summer day with two of his friends from school. The three of them decided to race the 70 yards out to the rope that marked the limit of the swimming area. When LE's two friends reached the rope, they looked around for LE but were unable to locate him. Panic-stricken, they waved their arms toward the beach to get the attention of the lifeguards. The two closest lifeguards spotted their distress signals, and after sounding their air horns, swam out to their location. A third lifeguard contacted the local fire department and then maneuvered a motorized rescue boat with basic emergency equipment out to them. After a few minutes of searching, one of the lifeguards found LE about 20 yards short of the rope. It was estimated that LE had been underwater for five minutes before being pulled to the surface and placed into the rescue boat. LE had a weak, slow pulse but had no respiratory efforts. One of the lifeguards initiated ventilation with a resuscitation mask with a one-way valve. By the time they arrived at the beach, EMS personnel were ready to assume responsibility for LE's care. They quickly intubated LE with a 7.5 mm endotracheal tube, suctioned the endotracheal tube, and transported him to the local emergency department while providing 100% oxygen via a bag-valve resuscitator. During the 12-minute transport, LE required defibrillation for two separate ventricular fibrillation events.

INITIAL ASSESSMENT

Age: 17-years-old
Height: 5' 9"
Weight: 185 lbs. (84 kg)
Heart Rate: 68 bpm
Respiratory Rate: 12 bpm (manual ventilation with bag-valve resuscitator)
Blood Pressure: 94/56 mm Hg
S_pO_2: 82% (100% O_2 via bag-valve resuscitator)
Temperature: 34.0° C
Breath Sounds: rhonchi (upper lobes), crackles and diminished (lower lobes)
Chest/Abdominal Inspection: normal
Cough/Sputum: suctioning required/large amounts of frothy, white secretions
Level of Consciousness: stuporous (no verbal response or eye opening to painful stimuli, but withdrew from pain)
Medical/Surgical History: none
Current Medications: none
Allergies: no known allergies

COMMENTS

Mechanical ventilation was initiated. Initial ventilator settings were: AC 16 500 mL 100% O_2 PEEP +10 cm H_2O. Heated normal saline intravenous fluids were started, and a warming blanket was used in an effort to correct LE's hypothermia.

DIAGNOSTIC RESULTS

ECG: sinus bradycardia with an occasional premature ventricular contraction (PVC)

Chest X-ray: tip of endotracheal tube 4 cm above carina, fluffy infiltrates throughout both lungs consistent with pulmonary edema, bibasilar pleural effusions and atelectasis

ABG: (AC 16 500 mL 100% O_2 PEEP +10 cm H_2O) (total respiratory rate = 16 bpm)
Hb = 13.6 g/dL
pH = 7.20
$PaCO_2$ = 30 mm Hg
PaO_2 = 160 mm Hg
SaO_2 = 100%
HCO_3^- = 11 mEq/L
BE = $^-$15 mEq/L
CaO_2 = 18.7 Vol%
Temperature = 34° C

ABG Interpretation: _____

Complete Blood Count:
White Blood Cells = 8.2 x $10^3/mm^3$
Red Blood Cells = 4.45 x $10^6/mm^3$
Hemoglobin = 13.8 g/dL
Hematocrit = 43.5%
Platelets = 380 x $10^3/mm^3$

Chemistry Profile:
Na^+ = 142 mEq/L
K^+ = 4.7 mEq/L
Cl^- = 107 mEq/L
CO_2 = 13 mEq/L
Glucose = 77 mg/dL
Blood Urea Nitrogen = 17 mg/dL
Creatinine = 0.8 mg/dL
Albumin = 4.0 g/dL
Mg^{2+} = 2.0 mg/dL

Ventilation Mechanics:
Plateau Pressure (P_{PLAT}): 38 cm H_2O
Static Lung Compliance (C_S): 18 mL/cm H_2O
Airway Resistance (R_{AW}): 15 cm H_2O/L/sec

COMMENTS
Ventilator settings were adjusted to: PC/AC 20/20 50% O_2 PEEP +10 cm H_2O T_I = 1.2 sec (titrate to keep exhaled tidal volume 450-500 mL).

INITIAL TREATMENT
furosemide 40 mg IV
heated normal saline IV fluids at 100 mL/hr
ceftriaxone sodium 1g IV
levofloxacin 750 mg IV

DIAGNOSTIC RESULTS
ABG: (PC/AC 20/20 50% O_2 PEEP +10 cm H_2O T_I = 1.2 sec) (exhaled tidal volume = 475 mL, total respiratory rate = 20 bpm)
Hb = 13.2 g/dL
pH = 7.28
$PaCO_2$ = 35 mm Hg
PaO_2 = 75 mm Hg
SaO_2 = 94%
HCO_3^- = 16 mEq/L
BE = $^-$10 mEq/L
CaO_2 = 16.9 Vol%
Temperature = 34.5° C

ABG Interpretation: _____

CASE DISCUSSION
1. What factors were in LE's favor in terms of survivability from this near drowning event?

2. What were some possible causes of this near drowning event?

3. What complications would the EMS personnel have anticipated when intubating LE?

4. What is the purpose of applying cricoid pressure during intubation? What are the hazards of applying cricoid pressure during intubation?

5. When manually ventilating an intubated patient with 100% oxygen via a bag-valve resuscitator, how can you improve oxygenation if a reliable S_pO_2 remains low, or if the S_pO_2 reading is unreliable and signs of hypoxemia/hypoxia exist?

6. List at least two reasons to question the reliability of the S_pO_2 reading obtained during the initial assessment in this case.

7. What is the likely cause of the acidosis identified in the ABG results?

8. Calculate the anion gap. What does the anion gap value indicate in this case?

9. List at least three possible causes for the development of ventricular fibrillation in this case.

10. Explain how pulmonary edema develops in a near drowning situation?

11. List the physiologic or structural changes responsible for the development of atelectasis in a near drowning event?

12. Do you agree with the initial ventilator settings?

13. What factor(s) prompted the change from volume ventilation to pressure control ventilation? Do you agree with the initial pressure control ventilation settings?

14. The ABG samples were temperature-corrected in this case. How are the pH, PaO_2, and $PaCO_2$ values of a sample affected when temperature-corrected for a hypothermic patient?

15. Locate at least two professional journal articles discussing the "alpha-stat" and "ph-stat" strategies for arterial blood gas management for hypothermic patients. Which strategy is recommended by the researcher(s) for each article?

16. What score would LE have received on the Glasgow Coma Scale?

17. What was the reasoning for the prophylactic treatment with broad spectrum antibiotics in this case?

18. How does the pathophysiological course differ between a near drowning in sea water and a near drowning in fresh water?

19. Explain the difference between a wet near drowning and a dry near drowning.

COMMENTS

LE's condition improved steadily, and he was able to be extubated within a 48-hour period. He had no identifiable neurological deficits, and his prognosis for a full recovery was excellent. Following extubation, LE stated that he just "ran out of gas" while swimming to the rope. He attributed his fatigue to the carrying of extra weight that he was working on to lose with the help of his parents and football coach. LE was discharged two days after extubation with instructions to complete the 14-day course of levofloxacin for pneumonia prophylaxis

CASE STUDY 14

LUNG CANCER

CASE INTRODUCTION
After persistent urgings from his wife, RF scheduled an appointment with his physician. For the previous two months, RF had experienced shortness of breath with exertion. Over the same time period, he also had a hacking, nonproductive cough that was occasionally productive with small amounts of blood-tinged sputum. A chest X-ray at RF's physician's office revealed a mass in the upper lobe of RF's right lung. RF was admitted to the local hospital for further evaluation.

INITIAL ASSESSMENT
Age: 54-years-old
Height: 6' 0"
Weight: 160 lbs. (73 kg)
Heart Rate: 108 bpm
Respiratory Rate: 24 bpm
Blood Pressure: 124/76 mm Hg
S$_p$O$_2$: 92% (room air)
Temperature: 37.0° C
Breath Sounds: clear (left upper lobe), crackles and diminished (right upper lobe), diminished (lower lobes)
Chest/Abdominal Inspection: normal
Cough/Sputum: fair, dry, nonproductive
Level of Consciousness: alert/oriented x 3
General Appearance/Behavior: anxious, annoyed about being in the hospital
Medical/Surgical History: none
Social History: smoker 1-2 PPD x 35 years
Current Medications: none
Allergies: no known allergies

DIAGNOSTIC RESULTS
Chest X-ray: COPD, well-defined large mass in right upper lobe, consolidation of right upper lobe

Chest CT: COPD, 4 cm mass in the central region of the right upper lobe, significant volume loss within right upper lobe

ABG: (room air)
Hb = 11.2 g/dL
pH = 7.37
$PaCO_2$ = 50 mm Hg
PaO_2 = 61 mm Hg
SaO_2 = 91%
HCO_3^- = 28 mEq/L
BE = 3 mEq/L
CaO_2 = 13.8 Vol%

ABG Interpretation: _____

Complete Blood Count:
White Blood Cells = 7.6 x $10^3/mm^3$
Red Blood Cells = 4.25 x $10^6/mm^3$
Hemoglobin = 11.5 g/dL
Hematocrit = 43.3%
Platelets = 280 x $10^3/mm^3$

Chemistry Profile:
Na^+ = 140 mEq/L
K^+ = 4.0 mEq/L
Cl^- = 103 mEq/L
CO_2 = 27 mEq/L
Glucose = 80 mg/dL
Blood Urea Nitrogen = 16 mg/dL
Creatinine = 0.7 mg/dL
Albumin = 4.1 g/dL
Mg^{2+} = 2.2 mg/dL

COMMENTS

RF's physician consulted a pulmonologist, and a bronchoscopy was performed. During the bronchoscopy, it was determined that a tumor had extended into the lobar bronchus of the right upper lobe. It was estimated that the lobar bronchus was 90% occluded by the tumor. Histology results of a tumor sample obtained by biopsy during the bronchoscopy concluded that the tumor was squamous cell carcinoma. Two days later, RF underwent surgery for a right upper lobe lobectomy. The thoracic surgeon's report stated that the right main stem bronchus, lymph nodes, visceral pleura, and chest wall showed no signs of invasion by the tumor, but the lung tissue surrounding the lobar bronchus, including the segmental bronchi, was involved. The ICU intensivist ordered a respiratory therapist evaluation for recommendations upon RF's admission to the ICU following the surgery.

ASSESSMENT
Heart Rate: 88 bpm
Respiratory Rate: 24 bpm
Blood Pressure: 110/65 mm Hg
S$_p$O$_2$: 93% (nasal cannula at 4 L/min)
Temperature: 37.6° C
Breath Sounds: wheezes and rhonchi (left upper lobe), diminished (lower lobes)
Chest/Abdominal Inspection: normal
Cough/Sputum: weak, congested, nonproductive
Level of Consciousness: lethargic
General Appearance/Behavior: lethargic, guarding right side
Medical/Surgical History: none
Social History: smoker 1-2 PPD x 35 years
Home Respiratory Medications: none
Home Oxygen: none
Home CPAP/NPPV: none
Allergies: no known allergies

DIAGNOSTIC RESULTS
ABG: (nasal cannula at 4 L/min)
Hb = 10.2 g/dL
pH = 7.35
PaCO$_2$ = 52 mm Hg
PaO$_2$ = 70 mm Hg
SaO$_2$ = 93%
HCO$_3$$^-$ = 28 mEq/L
BE = 2 mEq/L
CaO$_2$ = 12.9 Vol%

ABG Interpretation: _____

CASE DISCUSSION
1. Formulate an initial respiratory care plan that could have been used for RF post-operatively.

2. How does the mortality rate from lung cancer compare to other types of cancer in the United States?

3. List at least four factors relating to smoking that help to determine the risk of developing lung cancer.

4. Describe the lung cancer risks associated with passive smoking.

5. How are the terms "nodule" and "mass" defined?

6. What is the relative growth rate and metastatic tendencies of squamous cell carcinoma?

7. What evidence suggested that RF was likely to make a full recovery from the lung cancer?

8. How would the squamous cell carcinoma have been staged in this case?

9. What were the likely causes of RF's symptoms that prompted him to seek medical attention?

10. What is the relative growth rate and metastatic tendencies of small-cell (oat-cell) carcinoma?

11. How is small-cell carcinoma staged?

12. What is the general prognosis for patients with small-cell carcinoma?

13. What pathologic features distinguish adenocarcinoma from the other types of bronchogenic carcinoma?

14. What is the relative growth rate and metastatic tendencies of adenocarcinoma?

15. What is the relative growth rate and metastatic tendencies of large-cell carcinoma?

16. What is the superior vena cava syndrome? How can bronchogenic tumors cause the superior vena cava syndrome?

17. List the four commonly used treatment strategies for lung cancer.

18. RF had a chest tube inserted during surgery which was connected to a water seal chamber system. Bubbling was observed in the water seal chamber while the wall suction was on. What were the possible causes of the bubbling in the water seal chamber?

19. How is the location of an air leak determined when using a water seal chamber system?

20. What could bubbling in the water seal chamber indicate if the wall suction was turned off?

21. List two reasons why a chest tube would be clamped for a brief period of time.

22. What would be indicated if there was no bubbling in the water seal chamber 24-48 hours after the wall suction was turned off?

23. RF was discharged on the sixth day of his hospital admission. What recommendations for RF would you have offered to the discharging physician?

CASE STUDY 15

ADULT PNEUMONIA (TRACHEOSTOMY TUBE)

CASE INTRODUCTION

A "Respiratory STAT" was called by the emergency department staff at a local hospital. A 70-year-old patient with a tracheostomy tube experiencing respiratory distress was being transported to their facility by EMS personnel from the patient's home. The EMS radio report included information that the patient had a laryngectomy six months prior to this event as a result of laryngeal cancer. He was being transported with supplemental oxygen via a non-rebreathing mask at 15 L/min over his tracheostomy tube.

CASE DISCUSSION

1. How would you have prepared for the arrival of this patient?

INITIAL ASSESSMENT

Age: 70-years-old
Height: 5' 11"
Weight: 155 lbs. (70 kg)
Heart Rate: 120 bpm
Respiratory Rate: 36 bpm
Blood Pressure: 190/100 mm Hg
S_pO_2: 85% (non-rebreathing mask at 15 L/min)
Temperature: 39.6° C
Breath Sounds: severely diminished throughout all lung fields
Chest/Abdominal Inspection: decreased chest excursion bilaterally, inspiratory and accessory muscle use, abdominal paradox
Cough/Sputum: none
Level of Consciousness: alert/oriented x 3
General Appearance/Behavior: cyanotic, diaphoretic, obvious respiratory distress, mouthing the words "help me"

COMMENTS

During the rapid initial assessment, the tracheostomy tube was identified as a 6.0 mm uncuffed tracheostomy tube. Thick, dried secretions surrounded the opening of the tracheostomy tube, and no inner cannula was present.

CASE DISCUSSION

2. List the respiratory care interventions that you would have administered to this patient in the order that you would have administered them.

3. Considering your responses to the previous two case discussion questions, would you have been prepared to deliver the respiratory care interventions you had chosen for this patient?

4. If you were to assemble an emergency kit of some sort to be used for this type of scenario, what would you include in the kit?

INITIAL ASSESSMENT (ADDENDUM)

Medical/Surgical History: chronic obstructive pulmonary disease (COPD), laryngeal cancer, larygnectomy, hypertension

Social History: ex-smoker 1-2 PPD x 43 years (quit 5 years ago)

Current Medications: albuterol/ipratropium bromide, formoterol fumarate, losartan potassium

Allergies: cephalosporins

COMMENTS

Emergent respiratory care interventions were successful, and RC's condition stabilized without requiring immediate mechanical ventilation.

DIAGNOSTIC RESULTS

Chest X-ray: tracheostomy tube appropriately positioned in airway, COPD, multilobar infiltrates, bibasilar atelectasis

ABG: (F_1O_2 35%)
Hb = 12.2 g/dL
pH = 7.33
$PaCO_2$ = 60 mm Hg
PaO_2 = 68 mm Hg
SaO_2 = 92%
HCO_3^- = 31 mEq/L
BE = 5 mEq/L
CaO_2 = 15.2 Vol%

ABG Interpretation: _____

Complete Blood Count:
White Blood Cells = 17.2 x 10^3/mm^3
Red Blood Cells = 4.35 x 10^6/mm^3
Hemoglobin = 12.0 g/dL
Hematocrit = 39.8%
Platelets = 310 x 10^3/mm^3

Chemistry Profile:
Na^+ = 145 mEq/L
K^+ = 3.0 mEq/L
Cl^- = 104 mEq/L
CO_2 = 31 mEq/L
Glucose = 105 mg/dL
Blood Urea Nitrogen = 11 mg/dL
Creatinine = 0.4 mg/dL
Albumin = 3.0 g/dL
Mg^{2+} = 1.7 mg/dL

CASE DISCUSSION

5. How would you have administered the 35% supplemental oxygen to RC?

6. Were there any laboratory results that required intervention?

ASSESSMENT
Heart Rate: 92 bpm
Respiratory Rate: 20 bpm
Blood Pressure: 128/88 mm Hg
S_pO_2: 94% (F_IO_2 35%)
Temperature: 38.0° C
Breath Sounds: wheezes and rhonchi (upper lobes), diminished (lower lobes)
Chest/Abdominal Inspection: normal
Cough/Sputum: weak, congested, nonproductive
Level of Consciousness: alert/oriented x 3
General Appearance/Behavior: significant improvement since initial assessment, resting comfortably
Medical/Surgical History: chronic obstructive pulmonary disease (COPD), laryngeal cancer, larygnectomy, hypertension
Social History: ex-smoker 1-2 PPD x 43 years (quit 5 years ago)
Current Respiratory Medications: albuterol/ipratropium bromide aerosol treatments QID, formoterol fumarate 20 mcg/2 mL unit dose BID
Home Oxygen: none
Home CPAP/NPPV: none
Allergies: cephalosporins

CASE DISCUSSION
7. Formulate a respiratory care plan to be used for RC on admission to the ICU.

8. The ICU intensivist wrote an order for mechanical ventilation to be used overnight and requested ventilator setting recommendations from the respiratory therapist covering the ICU? What initial ventilator settings would you have recommended?

COMMENTS
During the night, RC experienced an episode of severe acute respiratory distress while receiving mechanical ventilatory support. The high pressure alarm was activated, and the exhaled tidal volumes were less than 100 mL. RC's heart rate had decreased to 45 bpm, and his S_pO_2 had decreased to 76%.

CASE DISCUSSION

9. What was the likely cause of the severe acute respiratory distress episode? How would you have corrected the situation?

10. Are there any changes that you would have made to your respiratory care plan, or other recommendations that you would have presented to the ICU intensivist, following the severe acute respiratory distress episode?

COMMENTS

RC responded well to the aggressive multidisciplinary care plan. Mechanical ventilatory support was discontinued after the second night. He was transferred to a medical/surgical unit on the morning of the third day, and supplemental oxygen was discontinued late on the fourth day. On the sixth day, he was transferred to an extended care facility for a period of two weeks and then returned home.

CASE DISCUSSION

11. Why would RC have had an uncuffed tracheostomy tube prior to this admission to the hospital?

12. Why are tenacious secretions, even in the absence of acute pulmonary infections, likely to be a recurring problem for patients with tracheostomy tubes or permanent stomas?

13. If a patient with a permanent stoma presented to the emergency department in severe respiratory distress, what emergent intervention(s) would you provide?

14. What is the best method for obtaining a sputum sample from a tracheostomy tube or permanent stoma to preserve the integrity of the specimen?

15. What would the presence of subcutaneous emphysema indicate when a tracheostomy tube is being used or is being inserted?

16. If a patient with a permanent stoma was in emergent need of an artificial airway and a tracheostomy tube was not immediately available, what would be the next best option?

17. What would massive airway bleeding indicate for a patient with a tracheostomy tube?

18. Why is it important to limit the movement of a patient following the initial surgical insertion of a tracheostomy tube?

19. How does a speaking valve allow a patient with a tracheostomy tube to talk?

20. What are the hazards of using a speaking valve with any kind of cuffed tracheostomy tube?

21. What are the advantages and disadvantages of using a fenestrated tracheostomy tube?

22. What is the ideal cuff pressure for an endotracheal tube or tracheostomy tube?